AUTOSOMAL DOMINANT DISORDERS

NEW RESEARCH

GENETICS - RESEARCH AND ISSUES

Additional books in this series can be found on Nova's website under the Series tab.

Additional E-books in this series can be found on Nova's website under the E-book tab.

AUTOSOMAL DOMINANT DISORDERS

NEW RESEARCH

PIETRO MARCIANO

AND

DENIS M. LANZA

EDITORS

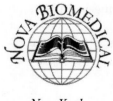

New York

Copyright © 2013 by Nova Science Publishers, Inc.

Library of Congress Cataloging-in-Publication Data

ISBN: 978-1-62808-760-4

Published by Nova Science Publishers, Inc. † New York

Contents

Preface

Autosomal dominant inheritance means an abnormal gene from one parent can cause disease, even though the matching gene from the other parent is normal. The abnormal gene dominates. In this book, the authors present new research in autosomal dominant disorders. Topics discussed include the pathophysiology and treatment of autosomal polycystic kidney disease; hereditary haemorrhagic telangiectasia or Rendu-Osler-Weber Syndrome; osteogenesis imperfecta; and autosomal dominant disorders associated with breast cancer.

Chapter 1 – Autosomal dominant polycystic kidney disease (ADPKD) is an inherited genetic disorder that results in progressive renal cyst formation and ultimately loss of renal function. Mutation in either *PKD1* or *PKD2*, which are the genes coding for polycystin-1 and polycystin-2, respectively, is the main cause of the disease. The mutation in *PKD1* accounts for 85% of all ADPKD cases, whereas only 15% of ADPKD cases result from *PKD2* mutations. ADPKD is a systemic disorder associated with cardiovascular, portal, pancreatic and gastrointestinal systems. ADPKD is a ciliopathy, a disease associated with abnormal primary cilia. Non-motile primary cilia, functioning as mechanosensory organelles, have been an intense research topic in ADPKD. It has been shown that both structural and functional defects in primary cilia result in cystic kidney and vascular hypertension. In particular, polycystin-1 and polycystin-2 are co-localized to primary cilia and are responsible for mechanosensory induced calcium influx in response to fluid-shear stress. Based on the multiple signaling pathways in ADPKD, different molecular targets have been developed for potential therapies.

Chapter 2 – Hereditary Haemorrhagic Telangiectasia (HHT) or Rendu Osler Weber syndrome (OMIM 187300/ORPHA774) is a vascular hereditary autosomic dominant multiorganic dysplasia,. Prevalence is in between 1 to 5,000/8,000 inhabitants around 65,000 in Europe, and 200,000 in USA); although due to founder effect, and insulation, it is higher in some regions as the Jura in France, Funen Island in Denmark and Caribbean Dutch Antilles where the prevalence may be 1 in 1,200 inhabitants. Diagnosis is based on the clinical criteria of Curaçao (Shovlin et al., 2000): epistaxis, telangiectases, first degree relative with HHT, and visceral arteriovenous malformations (AVMs), mainly in lung, liver and brain. For a positive diagnosis, 3 out of the 4 previous criteria are required. A positive genetic test implies also a positive diagnosis.

The clinical diagnosis requires then a detailed medical screening, with involvement of different medical specialities. Penetrance of the disease is variable increasing with age.

Pulmonary arteriovenous malformations (PAVMs) occur in aproximately 50% of patients, hepatic involvement in up to 70%, brain AVMs in 10% and spinal in 1%. However the most frequent clinical manifestation of HHT is epistaxis (nose bleeding) normally from light to moderate that affects 93% of patients and is present before the age of 21 in 90 % of cases (Faughnan et al., 2009).

The genetic origin of the disease is due to mutations of genes involved in the TGB-β pathway, critical for the normal development of blood vessels (Fernández et al. 2006). The first gene identified was *Endoglin (ENG)*, responsible for the 39-59% of the HHT cases (HHT 1); shortly after, *ALK1/(ACVRL1)* was discovered to be involved in 25-57% of cases (HHT2). In around 2% of the HHT patients, the mutation is located in the *MADH4/Smad4* gene leading to a combined syndrome of Juvenile Polyposis and HHT (JPHT). A third and a fourth locus have been mapped on chromosomes 5 and 7 with no genes identified at the moment. Endoglin plays a key role in vasculogenesis and arterial/venous differentiation in embryos, as well as in angiogenesis and neovascularization processes in the adult; ALK1 is responsible for the events occurring during the activation phase of angiogenesis. Haploinsufficiency is accepted as the mechanism of pathogenicity for the HHT.

Chapter 3 – Osteogenesis imperfecta is the most common heritable cause of fractures in children. It is not a single disorder but a large group of diseases most, but not all, being caused by defects of the genes coding for collagen. Autosomal dominant inheritance is the most common finding in familial cases but new mutations occur. Autosomal recessive inheritance does occur and mosaicism is recognized.

The great molecular heterogeneity is reflected in great clinical and radiological variation. Some cases are so severe that survival beyond intra-uterine life is impossible. At the other extreme some patients, undoubtedly affected their family history, have few fractures and live normal lives. Fractures often occur spontaneously and previously asymptomatic fractures in various stages of healing are often found radiologically. While most symptomatic fractures are diaphyseal, all types of fractures including metaphyseal fractures, rib fractures and skull fractures do occur.

Modern management involves good orthopaedic surgery; it is particularly important to avoid prolonged immobilisation of limbs to avoid superimposed osteopenia. Drug therapy, particularly with pamidronate, may be appropriate in children with the more severe forms of the disorder. Specific attention may be needed to scoliosis, basilar invagination or deafness. Good occupational therapy to maximise mobility is important. Children with osteogenesis imperfecta have normal intelligence and good education is vital.

Chapter 4 – The sudden rise of new biochemical and molecular techniques, have enabled a better understanding of the physiological and biochemical bases of the tumorogenesis, leaving clear that cancer is a "*genetic condition*". Breast cancer is one of the most common cancers in women, affecting one in six women among 40-59 years in the world; so it has been widely studied. Unlike the majority of genetic diseases, in which the presence of a mutation in a particular gene is sufficient for delineation of a phenotype (monogenic); in breast cancer, the simple presence of a mutation in a particular gene is not enough to explain it. Approximately 90% of breast cancer cases occur sporadically and the majority of cases are caused by mutations in the *BRCA1* or *BRCA2* gene. However, in 5-10% of cases of breast cancer has been identify an autosomal dominant transmission, as well as mutations in specific genes such as *TP53, PTEN, CHECK2 STK11* among others, that considerably increase the susceptibility to this condition. Autosomal dominant transmission of this disease has opened a new chapter in cancer medicine since the presence of any of these mutations in a patient, forces the doctor to carry out a deep investigation of the condition in order to establish a prognosis, as well as effective strategies for survival and family prevention. This chapter makes a brief revision of the autosomal dominat disorders Li-Fraumani syndrome, Cowden Disease and Peutz-Jeghers syndrome, which have a high susceptibility to development of breast cancer.

In: Autosomal Dominant Disorders   ISBN: 978-1-62808-760-4
Editors: P. Marciano and D. M. Lanza © 2013 Nova Science Publishers, Inc.

Chapter 1

Autosomal Dominant Polycystic Kidney Disease: Pathophysiology and Treatment

Ashraf M. Mohieldin[1], Viralkumar S. Upadhyay[2],
Albert C. M. Ong[3] and Surya M. Nauli[1,2]*
[1]Department of Medicinal and Biological Chemistry,
The University of Toledo, Toledo, Ohio, US
[2]Department of Pharmacology, The University of Toledo,
Toledo, Ohio, US
[3]Academic Unit of Nephrology, University of Sheffield Medical School,
Sheffield, UK

Abstract

Autosomal dominant polycystic kidney disease (ADPKD) is an inherited genetic disorder that results in progressive renal cyst formation and ultimately loss of renal function. Mutation in either *PKD1* or *PKD2*, which are the genes coding for polycystin-1 and polycystin-2, respectively, is the main cause of the disease. The mutation in *PKD1*

* Corresponding author: Surya M. Nauli, Ph.D., The University of Toledo, Department of Pharmacology; MS 1015, Health Education building; Room 274, 3000 Arlington Ave, Toledo, OH 43614, Phone: 419-383-1910, Fax: 419-383-1909, Email: Surya.Nauli@UToledo.Edu.

accounts for 85% of all ADPKD cases, whereas only 15% of ADPKD cases result from *PKD2* mutations. ADPKD is a systemic disorder associated with cardiovascular, portal, pancreatic and gastrointestinal systems. ADPKD is a ciliopathy, a disease associated with abnormal primary cilia. Non-motile primary cilia, functioning as mechanosensory organelles, have been an intense research topic in ADPKD. It has been shown that both structural and functional defects in primary cilia result in cystic kidney and vascular hypertension. In particular, polycystin-1 and polycystin-2 are co-localized to primary cilia and are responsible for mechanosensory induced calcium influx in response to fluid-shear stress. Based on the multiple signaling pathways in ADPKD, different molecular targets have been developed for potential therapies.

1. Introduction

Polycystic kidney disease (PKD) is a group of renal cyst diseases that are characterized by the formation of fluid-filled cysts. PKD is classified into acquired and hereditary forms. The acquired form of polycystic kidney disease is characterized by long standing chronic renal failure and subsequent dialysis. However, most forms of polycystic kidney disease are hereditary, including nephronophthisis and medullary cystic kidney diseases. The most common hereditary forms of PKD are autosomal dominant PKD (ADPKD) and autosomal recessive PKD (ARPKD). The pathophysiological presentation of these diseases starts from birth in ARPKD and in the adult years in ADPKD. While the key feature of ARPKD is elongated cysts due to collecting duct dilatation, the hallmark of ADPKD is large focal cysts arising from the rapidly dividing tubular epithelial cells. An important difference between the two is that cysts in ADPKD become isolated, while cysts remain in contact with their tubular origin in ARPKD [1].

The estimated prevalence of ADPKD is one in every 500 to 1,000 individuals [2, 3]. ADPKD is caused by mutation in either *PKD1* or *PKD2*, encoding polycystin-1 or polycystin-2, respectively [4-6]. Mutations in *PKD1* are responsible for more than 85% of ADPKD whereas mutations in *PKD2* account for 15%. On the other hand, ARPKD is caused by mutations in *PKHD1* gene, with a prevalence of one in 20,000 live births [7].

In ADPKD, cysts can form not only in the kidney but also in other organs such as the liver, seminal vesicles, pancreas, and arachnoid membrane [8-10]. Clinically, ADPKD is also characterized by vascular abnormalities such as intracranial aneurysms, dilatation of the aortic root, dissection of the aortic thoracic aorta, mitral valve prolapse, and abdominal wall hernias. Imaging studies are primarily used to diagnose ADPKD. Magnetic resonance imaging (MRI) is used to determine kidney volume as well as to exclude intracranial aneurysms, particularly in patients at high risk. Genetic testing is clinically available for both *PKD1* and *PKD2*.

2. Primary Cilia and Cystic Kidney

Primary cilia are found on almost all mammalian cell types including renal epithelia where they act as mechanosensory organelles, sensing and responding to urinary flow in the nephron [11, 12]. Previous studies have showed that primary cilia contain polycystin-1 and polycystin-2 [11-13]. Polycystin-1 and polycystin-2 are glycoproteins widely expressed in various tissues, including renal epithelia, vascular endothelia and cardiac myocytes. Polycystin-1, with 11 transmembrane domains, is developmentally regulated [14, 15]. Subcellular localization of polycystin-1 seems to depend on the stage of development and cell polarization of the tubular epithelium [16, 17]. Polycystin-2 is a calcium channel with six transmembrane domains [6, 18]. The transmembrane region of polycystin-2 is homologous to polycystin-1, voltage-activated and transient receptor potential (TRP) channel subunits [19].

Ultrastructurally, the cilium is a hair-like structure filled with microtubules and enclosed by the ciliary membrane. Primary cilia contains the outer nine microtubule doublets, but lack the inner pair of microtubules, and that is why it is known as a "9+0" axoneme. The outer microtubule doublet is connected by a structural protein nexin to form a ring in the primary cilium [20]. The basal body or mother centriole is a region in which doublet microtubules rise from the triplet microtubules and is known as the transition zone. The basal body and centriole join together and form a centrosome, which serves as the cell's main microtubule organization. The ciliary necklace, which is made of a series of membrane proteins at the transition zone, helps differentiate the ciliary membrane from the cell's plasma membrane [21]. The primary cilium also has ciliary pockets on each side of the plasma membrane [22]. These are invaginations into the cell membrane adjacent to the ciliary necklace common to many species. The semi-enclosed area is created by apertures at the transition zone, known as the ciliary sheath, and is thought to restrict protein and lipid entry into the cilium; this area is formed during ciliogenesis [23, 24].

Within an epithelial cilium, the polycystin complex has been proposed to have a role in sensing and mediating flow dependent mechanosensory calcium signaling [11, 12, 25-28]. The involvement of polycystins in primary cilia has further provided that ciliary dysfunction results in abnormal planar cell polarity [29, 30].

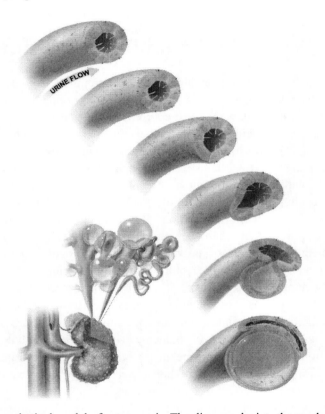

Figure 1. Hypothetical model of cytogenesis. The diagram depicts the mechanosensory function of a renal tubular cilium and how cilia dysfunction can lead to cyst formation. The cilium plays an important role as a mechanosensory organelle that transmits extracellular signals such as urine and blood flow into the cell. These signals may provide critical messages to the cell regarding the direction of cell division along the tubule. A mutation in either *PKD1* and/or *PKD2* will result in ciliary dysfunction in sensing fluid movement. The abnormality in ciliary sensing could result in the loss of many signals, including those regulating planar cell polarity. As a result, the direction of cell division becomes randomized, resulting in increased tubular diameter rather than tubular elongation. Consequently, cyst growth will occur in isolated focal manner along the renal tubules. More cysts illustrated from the neighboring nephrons are depicted on the bottom left corner. The diagram was modified from the original [152].

Within the kidney anatomy, planar cell polarity is defined as an organized arrangement of cells in a plane of tissue perpendicular to the apical-basal axis as a direction for the orientation of cell division. Using cystic kidney mouse models, defects in cilia function have been shown to cause abnormal spindle pole orientation during cell division [31]. It is therefore thought that inactivation of ciliary protein would result in abnormal planar cell polarity, which in turn triggers an increase in renal tubular diameter. It is hypothesized that the net result is the initiation of cyst formation (Figure 1).

3. Liver Cysts

The most common extrarenal manifestation of ADPKD is the formation of liver cysts, the severity and frequency of which increase with age. Polycystic liver also occurs as a genetically distinct disease in the absence of renal cysts. The prevalence of liver cysts is between 75 to 90% among ADPKD patients [32]. Their prevalence by magnetic resonance imaging is 58% in patients 15 to 24 years old, 85% in 25- to 34-year-olds, and 94% in 35- to 46-year-old subjects [33]. Hepatic cysts are more prevalent and cyst volumes larger in women than in men [34]. In addition, women who have had multiple pregnancies or have used oral contraceptive drugs or estrogen replacement therapy have worse disease outcomes suggesting an estrogen effect on hepatic cyst growth.

4. Pancreatic Cysts

The pancreas, involved in secretion of hormones and gastric enzymes, contains a maze of tubules and ducts involved in carrying the enzymes to the intestinal lumen. Ductal epithelial cells secrete bicarbonate to neutralize the acidic chime from the stomach [35]. True congenital cysts of the pancreas are rare. Multiple congenital pancreatic cysts are mostly associated with ADPKD, although they are also found in cystic fibrosis, von Hippel-Lindau disease, Ivemark syndrome, and Meckel Gruber syndrome [36]. In the case of ADPKD, a connection between cilia defects and pancreatic pathologies suggested a link with pancreatic lesions. In some cases, remnants of chronic pancreatitis are found in approximately 10% of patients with ADPKD [37, 38]. In addition, other studies in mutant mice with defects in cilia formation have shown several pancreatic abnormalities, including exocrine cell atrophy, ductal dilation, and collagen deposition [39, 40]. Moreover, another mutant mouse study demonstrated that the absence of cilia in pancreatic cells produces pancreatic lesions that resemble those found in patients with chronic pancreatitis or cystic fibrosis [41].

5. Diverticulitis

Patients with ESRD due to ADPKD have a higher prevalence (20%) of colon diverticulitis than do those with ESRD due to other etiologies (3%) [41]. Not only do ADPKD-ESRD patients have a higher incidence of diverticulitis, they also have a higher complication rate associated with colon diverticulitis [42]. Colon perforation, fistula formation, intra-abdominal abscess, and generalized peritonitis are frequently diagnosed in ADPKD patients [43, 44]. However, colonic diverticula are usually asymptomatic. Major complications of diverticulitis, including perforation-related peritonitis, sepsis and shock, occur in only a small percentage of patients.

6. Pain

Pain is the most frequent complaint among ADPKD patients. A recent study of 171 ADPKD patients reported that 71.3% of the patients had lower back pain, the most common site of pain in this group [45]. About 30% of this group had radiculopathy symptoms. The second most common site for pain was reported to be the abdominen. Abdominal pain was reported by 61% of ADPKD patients. The character of pain described by these patients varied from a dull ache (49.5%), uncomfortable fullness (42.7%), stabbing pain (40.4%), and cramping pain (33.0%). Chronic headache and chest pain were also reported in these patients. Pain in ADPKD can occur acutely or persist becoming chronic. Cyst rupture or hemorrhage, infected cysts and renal stones are considered the most common phases of acute pain [32]. Progressive kidney enlargement may cause dull, chronic pain by stretching of the renal capsule. Larger renal volumes accompanied by asymmetric, hypertrophic lumbosacral muscle spasm are likely to be the basis of chronic back pain.

7. Hypertension

With the availability of renal replacement therapies for patients reaching ESRD, cardiovascular complications have emerged as the major cause of death in patients with ADPKD [46, 47]. Hypertension is diagnosed in 50–70% of patients usually before any substantial reduction in glomerular filtration rate is observed [48]. Hypertension relates to progressive kidney enlargement and to ESRD, but in some studies has been reported to be an independent risk factor for progression to ESRD [49]. In addition, hypertension occurs at a much earlier age in ADPKD patients than in the general population [50]. About 10-20% of children with ADPKD develop hypertension, and the majority of adults are hypertensive before any loss of kidney function. The median age for diagnosis of hypertension in ADPKD was 32 years for males and 34 years for females, compared to a median age of 45-55 years in patients with essential hypertension [50, 51]. Not surprisingly, the occurrence of hypertension is greater in both male and female ADPKD patients when their affected parents are hypertensive [32]. The pathogenesis of hypertension in ADPKD patients is complex and multifactorial [52].

7.1. Endothelin

Endothelin-1 (ET-1) has been reported to exert multiple effects on renal physiology [53]. In addition, there is good evidence that many renal cell types, including tubular cells, synthesize and are affected by ET-1, indicating its role as an autocrine or a paracrine factor [54, 55]. ET-1 has also been demonstrated to play a significant role in human renal tubular cells, and it can stimulate collagen I gene expression in human renal interstitial fibroblasts [56, 57]. Moreover, tubular cell proliferation has been reported to be an early feature of precystic tubules in human ADPKD and many rodent PKD models [58].

Several studies have shown that patients with ADPKD have high expression of ET-1 in the renal cystic epithelium [57, 59]. ET-1 is also found to be present in cyst fluid [60]. Another study demonstrated that patients with ADPKD have increased plasma levels of ET-1 compared with healthy controls and patients with essential hypertension [61]. Moreover, endothelium-dependent relaxation is impaired and endothelial nitric oxide synthase activity is decreased in normotensive patients with ADPKD [62]. These alterations cause up-regulation of ET-1 and dysfunction of the NO system, resulting in arterial vasoconstriction [63].

Other studies have demonstrated a physiological role for ET-1 acting via tubular ET_B receptor to regulate sodium and water excretion in kidney collecting ducts [64, 65]. Activation of tubular ET_B receptors inhibits vasopressin action, thereby promoting diuresis and sodium excretion by inhibiting Na^+/K^+ ATPase and /or epithelial sodium channels [66]. As a result, ET_B inhibition can potentiate vasopressin action in cysts derived from the collecting duct and consequently stimulate cyst growth [67, 68]. It is also noteworthy that the increased sympathetic activity and circulating ET-1 levels could result from the stimulation of intrarenal renin-angiotensin-aldosterone system due to progressive cyst enlargement, thereby leading to systemic hypertension [69].

7.2. Primary Cilia and Nitric Oxide

Primary cilia regulated nitric oxide (NO) production play an important role in the regulation of vascular tone [70, 71]. In a blood vessel, an abrupt increase in blood pressure or shear stress can be detected by mechanosensory proteins localized in the cilia [72, 73]. Extracellular fluid mechanics can then be transduced and translated into a complex of intracellular signaling, which in turn activates endothelial nitric oxide synthase (eNOS), an endothelial enzyme that synthesizes NO. The released NO diffuses from endothelial cells to neighboring smooth muscle cells, thus promoting vasodilation.

Both polycystin-1 and polycystin-2 are expressed in the endothelial and vascular smooth muscle cells of all major vessels [74, 75]. Mutations in both *PKD1* and *PKD2* have been shown to contribute to hypertension [76, 77], in part by the failure to convert an increase in mechanical blood flow into cellular NO biosynthesis [72, 73]. It has been shown that impaired endothelial dependent relaxation from aorta cells of *PKD1* knockout mice, due to a defect in (NO) release from the endothelium (Figure 2), correlates with a decrease in Ca^{2+} dependent endothelial NO synthesis activity [78]. We also previously reported the loss of response to fluid-shear stress in mouse endothelial cells with knockdown or knockout of *PKD2* [72]. In addition to the mouse data, polycystin-2 null endothelial cells generated from *PKD2* patients that do not show polycystin-2 in the cilia are unable to sense fluid flow. This further indicates that overall major effect of endothelial cilia function is to decrease total peripheral resistance, thereby lowering the blood pressure through the production of NO.

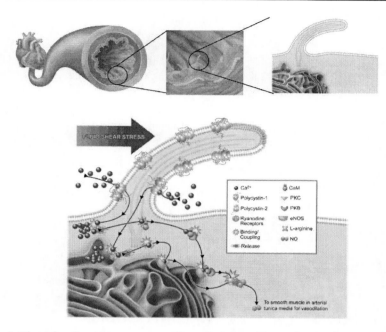

Figure 2. The role of mechanosensory cilia and nitric oxide production in ADPKD. The biochemical production and release of nitric oxide (NO) is dependant on the function of endothelial cilia in the vasculature. In ADPKD, dysfunctional cilia are not able to mechanically sense blood flow, and NO is not produced, resulting in increased blood pressure. The bending of cilia by fluid-shear stress activates the mechanosensory polycystins complex and initiates biochemical synthesis and release of NO. This biochemical cascade involves extracellular calcium influx (Ca^{2+}), followed by the activation of various calcium-dependent proteins including calmodulin (CaM), protein kinase C (PKC) andAkt/PKB). This illustration was modified from the original [153].

A final contributor to loss of vascular tone regulation could be reduction in NO bioavailability secondary to increased reactive oxygen species at least in *PKD2* heterozygous smooth muscle cells [79].

7.3. Angiotensin

Changes in renal structure may play an important role in the pathogenesis of hypertension in ADPKD patients (Figure 3). Cyst enlargement in ADPKD is associated with medial vascular changes and compression of the adjacent parenchyma with resultant areas of renal ischemia and activation of the renin-angiotensin-aldosterone system (RAAS).

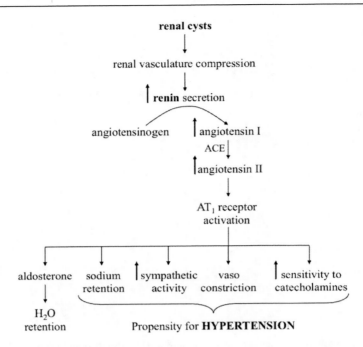

Figure 3. RAAS regulation in ADPKD. Renal cysts compress and disrupt the vascular network in the kidney, which leads to ischemic kidney. It was proposed that this would increase the release of renin from the juxtaglomerular apparatus. The increase in renin secretion would eventually accelerate the conversion of angiotensinogen to angiotensin I, which is further converted by angiotensin-converting enzyme (ACE) to angiotensin II. As a result, the angiotensin receptor (AT1) is activated initiating cascades of responses resulting in hypertension. This illustration was modified from the original [154].

In support of this, hypertensive patients with ADPKD demonstrate significantly greater renal volumes than patients with normal blood pressure [32, 80]. Other components of the RAAS, including angiotensinogen, angiotensin converting enzyme (ACE), angiotensin II receptor and angiotensin II peptide, have also been detected in cysts and dilated tubules in ADPKD kidneys [81]. Activation of the RAAS has been found in normotensive and hypertensive PKD patients, regardless of their blood pressure and renal function [82]. Not surprisingly, the high levels of circulating angiotensin II in PKD patients have been shown to contribute to the development of vascular hypertrophy, which is further implicated in vascular remodeling [83]. In addition, changes in the vasculature during the course of the PKD progression have been observed in both human [84, 85] and animal studies [86, 87].

Increased sympathetic activity has been reported in hypertensive patients with ADPKD, regardless of renal function [88, 89], suggesting that sympathetic hyperactivity could contribute to the pathogenesis of hypertension in ADPKD patients. ACE-I ramipril and the beta-blocker metoprolol are both effective as first-line therapies in hypertensive PKD patients [90]. It is recommended that more aggressive blood pressure control with these agents is necessary in order to be beneficial for ADPKD patients [32]. It should be noted that angiotensin can stimulate the sympathetic nervous system and vice-versa.

8. Left Ventricular Hypertrophy

Left ventricular hypertrophy (LVH) is well known as a powerful independent risk factor for cardiovascular morbidity and mortality [91]. Increased left ventricular mass index (LVMI) is associated with worse renal and patient outcomes in ADPKD [92]. Chapman and colleagues further reported in their study that LVH was found in 48% of hypertensive subjects with ADPKD [93]. Their study also showed a significant correlation between hypertension and LVMI, which has been demonstrated in both children and adults with ADPKD. In addition, children whose blood pressure was within the upper quartile of the normal range were found to have a significantly greater LVMI than those with lower blood pressure [94].

Bardaji and colleagues showed that young normotensive ADPKD patients and preserved renal function had increased LVMIs and Doppler abnormalities consistent with early diastolic dysfunction in a cross-sectional study of three different groups of ADPKD patients [95]. Another study by Oflaz and colleagues showed that biventricular diastolic dysfunction was present in both hypertensive and normotensive ADPKD patients with well-preserved renal function [96]. Verdecchia et al. reported that hypertensive patients whose nocturnal blood pressure remains elevated demonstrate higher LVMI compared to those whose blood pressure falls at night [97]. Furthermore, Li Kam et al. demonstrated that hypertensive patients with ADPKD who have normal renal function or mild renal impairment have significantly lower nocturnal decreases in blood pressure compared to patients with essential hypertension [98]. Another study has shown that the nocturnal fall in blood pressure was attenuated even in young normotensive ADPKD patients [99]. In this study, a higher LVMI was closely related to the ambulatory systolic blood pressure in normotensive patients. It has also been shown that insulin resistance is significantly associated with LVMI in healthy relatives and patients with *PKD1* mutations independent of other factors known to increase LVMI such as age, body weight, systolic blood pressure and albuminuria [100]. Thus, the stimulation of angiotensin II and the sympathetic nervous system due to hyperinsulinemia may contribute to increased LVMI in *PKD1* patients [100, 101]. However, other factors besides hypertension, including anemia, obesity, and sodium intake, as well as increased activity of the renin-angiotensin-aldosterone system and other genetic factors, may be associated with LVH, in both hypertensive and normotensive ADPKD patients [93]. The etiology of LVH is likely to be multifactorial but hypertension still plays a major role in its development [102].

9. Aneurysm

ADPKD patients have a higher prevalence (4.0-11.7%) of intracranial aneurysms than the general population (1.0%) [103, 104]. In addition, four to seven percent of patients with ADPKD die from intracranial aneurysm rupture, and such deaths occur at a younger age than in sporadic cases [105]. Intracranial aneurysm rupture seems to be more common in certain families with ADPKD [106, 107]. This indicates that a family history can be an important tool in assessing the risk of aneurysm rupture in ADPKD. Extracranial aneurysm, such as in coronary arteries, abdominal aorta, renal artery and splenic artery, has been reported in ADPKD patients suggesting that these are primary abnormalities [108, 109]. Other potential cardiovascular features reported in patients with ADPKD include biventricular diastolic dysfunction, endothelial dysfunction, increased carotid intima-media thickness, impaired coronary flow and cardiac valvular defects.

10. Therapeutic Treatments for Cardiovascular Complications

Early and effective treatment of hypertension is highly recommended for the prevention of cardiovascular complications in ADPKD patients. Since LVH and hypertension contribute significantly to cardiovascular morbidity and mortality, controlling these factors can positively impact patient health and sruvival. Antihypertensive treatment with an ACE inhibitor has been shown to reverse LVH over a seven-year follow-up period, thus decreasing an important risk factor for cardiovascular death in ADPKD patients [110]. A seven-year prospective, randomized study in 75 hypertensive patients with ADPKD and LVH compared the effects of rigorous and standard blood pressure control (<120/80 mmHg versus 135–140/85–90 mmHg) on LVH and renal function. Ecder and Schrier suggest that both strategies decreased LVH significantly [46]. In addition, rigorous blood pressure control was considerably more effective in decreasing LVMI than was standard blood pressure control. More patients in the rigorous-control group (71%) achieved normal LVMI than in the standard group (44%). A subgroup analysis showed that patients who received the ACE inhibitor enalapril experienced a significantly greater decrease in LVH than patients who received the calcium-channel blocker amlodipine, despite similar blood pressure control. On this basis, a blood pressure goal of less than 120/80 mmHg has been recommended that patients with ADPKD with hypertension and LVH [46].

11. Modern Therapies to Halt Progression of Renal Cysts

Since ADPKD accounts for up to 10% of patients on renal replacement therapy, an effective disease-modifying drug would have significant implications. The identification of *PKD1* and *PKD2* has led to an explosion in knowledge identifying new disease mechanisms and testing new drugs. Currently, there are three major treatment strategies to treat or reduce progression of kidney failure in ADPKD: to reduce cAMP levels, inhibit cell proliferation, and reduce fluid secretion [111, 112].

11.1. cAMP

Cyclic AMP (cAMP) elevation has an inhibitory effect on cell growth in normal kidney epithelial cells, while it stimulates cell proliferation in ADPKD cells [113]. The molecular basis of this may be Protein kinase-A activation of the B-Raf/MEK/ERK signaling pathway [114]. It has also been proposed that hyper-phosphorylation of polycystin-2 by protein kinase-A can contribute to cystic kidney formation by loss of PC2 inhibition of cell cycle progression [115]. Elevated cAMP also results in increased fluid secretion and cyst enlargement by stimulating the apical CFTR channel and specific basolateral transporters [114, 116]. Vasopressin V2 receptor (V2R) is a major regulator of cAMP production and adenylyl cyclase activity in the principal cells lining the collecting ducts [116]. Nagao et al. showed that high water intake can suppress vasopressin and decrease cyst and renal volumes in PCK rats, with a reduced activity of the cAMP dependent B-Raf/MEK/ERK pathway [117]. The strongest evidence for a pathogenic role of vasopressin in cyst growth comes from a study which demonstrated that deletion of vasopressin in PCK rats by breeding these with Brattleboro rats results in lower renal cAMP levels and near complete inhibition of cystogenesis [118]. The V2R antagonist OPC-31260 substantially reduced cAMP concentrations and inhibited cyst development in several rodent cystic kidney models [119-121]. Tolvaptan, an analogue with higher potency and selectivity for the human V2R, was equally effective in reducing renal cysts in PCK rats [122]. In a recently concluded phase III clinical trial, Tolvaptan slowed the increase in total kidney volume and the decline in GFR over a three-year period in patients with ADPKD [123]. There was however a significant drop-out rate in the treated group and a few patients developed liver enzyme abnormalities which reversed on cessation of treatment. It is worth mentioning that these drugs had no effect on liver cysts, due to the absence of VPV2R in the liver [34].

11.2. mTOR

The mTOR pathway was shown to be directly regulated by primary cilia [124]. In addition, mTOR signaling can be regulated by different signaling inputs and leads to changes in activity of many cellular processes that drive cyst growth [125]. The polycystin-1 protein directly interacts with the Tuberous Sclerosis Complex-2 (TSC2) protein. TSC2 and Tuberous Sclerosis Complex-1 (TSC1) protein are normally found together in a complex. Bonnet et al. demonstrated that combined mutations in *PKD1* and either *Tsc1* or *Tsc2* in compound heterozygous mice was associated with a more severe renal cystic phenotype than in mice with either mutation alone [126]. mTOR activity is regulated by TSC1-TSC2 complex through several cellular inputs [124, 127]. Thereafter, mTOR regulates protein synthesis, lipid biosynthesis, hypoxia response, *de novo* ceramide synthesis, PKC, AKT, fluid secretion, glycosphingolipid metabolism and ion balance, all of which are dysregulated in PKD. Particularly, the activity of mTORC1, mTORC2, PKC, AKT, ERK, IGF-1, CFTR and EGF-1 are all increased in ADPKD patients [124]. It has therefore been proposed that mTOR inhibition can delay cystic growth and expansion in ADPKD kidneys. More specifically, mTOR kinase activity is aberrantly increased in ADPKD patients [128]. Treatments with mTOR inhibitor, such as rapamycin, sirolimus or everolimus, decrease renal cyst size and improve kidney function in cystic kidney models [129, 130] although not in humans [131, 132].

11.3. EGFR

Members of the epidermal growth factor (EGF)-family bind to ErbB (EGFR)-family receptors, which play an important role in the regulation of various fundamental cell processes including cell proliferation and differentiation [133]. Although ErbB2 and ErbB4 have been detected in developing ureteric buds, EGFR is the predominant ErbB receptor expressed in normal adult mammalian kidney tubules [134, 135]. In addition, EGF-ErbB receptor-mediated interaction is a key element in renal tubular cell proliferation, not only in normal kidneys but also in cyst formation and enlargement. EGF is a well-known mitogen for normal renal epithelia and has been shown to stimulate hyperproliferation in renal cystic epithelia [136, 137]. As mentioned above, EGF and EGF-immunoreactive peptide species are secreted into the apical medium of cultured ADPKD epithelia, and high mitogenic concentrations of EGF have been measured in ADPKD cyst fluids [1]. Interestingly, the increase of EGF-1 can result in ERK activation through Ras and (B-Raf) Raf signaling pathways, which could in turn regulate the TSC1-TSC2 complex in ADPKD patients [125]. Administration of EGFR inhibitors, such as EKI-785 and EKB-569, in some renal cystic models decreases kidney weights and cyst volumes, suggesting a therapeutic potential of EGFR inhibition in ADPKD treatment [138]. In addition, EGF-like growth factors such as TGF-α and heparin-binding EGF have been found to be abnormally expressed in human ADPKD epithelial cells [133, 139].

11.4. Other Potential Targets

Besides cAMP, mTOR and EGF, there are other potential drugs targeting other signaling pathways such as SR, AP-1, c-Src, Raf, MEK, ERK, A3AR, CFTR and IGF-1 [113, 125], all of which are abnormally regulated in patients with ADPKD (Figure 4). A number of drugs showing promise in preclinical models have been or are being tested in clinical trials (Table 1).

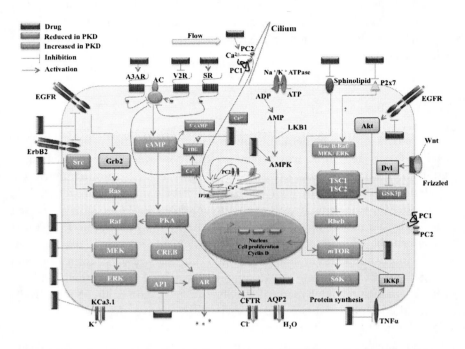

Figure 4. The signaling pathway and drug targets in ADPKD cystic cells. The diagram illustrates the mechanism that polycystin-1 (PC1), polycystin-2 (PC2), signaling proteins, molecules, receptors and drugs exert on signaling pathways leading to cyst formation. The green box indicates drug targets proposed for ADPKD. The blue box indicates the reduced molecules and signaling proteins in ADKPD. The orange box indicates the increased signaling proteins in ADPKD, which are thought to be responsible for an increase in cell proliferation including cAMP, EGFR, Ras/Raf/ERK, Src, CFTR, AC, and mTOR activity. In addition, EGFR activation is also enhanced by amphiregulin (AR) that is abnormally expressed in cystic cells through cAMP, CREB and AP1 signaling. Furthermore, altered EGFR and cAMP signaling stimulate mTOR activity by activation of Akt and Ras/Raf/ERK, which inhibit the TSC1/TSC2 complex. The sphingolipid, Na$^+$/K$^+$ ATPase, Wnt and P2x7 purinergic receptors are also involved in the regulation of mTOR activity. Na$^+$/K$^+$ ATPase also regulates the KCa3.1 receptor. However, the abnormal cAMP accumulation contributes to the activation of the Ras/Raf/ERK signaling pathway directly or by the activation of Src, which is able to interact with EGFR in its EGFR/ErbB2 heterodimer form. Other receptors that are involved in ADPKD include adenosine receptor-3A (A3AR), vasopressin receptor-2 (V2R) and somatostatin receptor (SR), which regulate activity of adenylate cyclase (AC). This illustration was adapted from the original [112].

Table 1. Current clinical trials in ADPKD

	Drugs	Signaling pathway	Study design	Treatment duration (months)	Clinical phase trial	Clinical trial status	Clinical trials Gov. identifier	Ref.
1	Octreotide	Analogue of somatostatin known to inhibit cAMP pathway in ADKPD and ADPLD	Randomized, double-blind, Placebo controlled and crossover	12	phase 2/3	Completed /failed	NCT00426153	[140, 141]31
2	Lanreotide	Analogue of somatostatin known to inhibit cAMP pathway in ADKPD and ADPLD	Randomized, double-blind and placebo controlled	6	phase 2/3	Completed	NCT00565097	[142]
3	Sirolimus	mTOR inhibitor	Randomized and penlabel	18	phase 2/3	Completed/ failed	NCT00346918	[132]
4	Sirolimus (SIRENA study)	mTOR inhibitor	Randomized, open-label and crossover	6	phase 2	Completed	NCT00491517	[143]
5	Everolimus	mTOR inhibitor	Multicenter, randomized, double-blind, placebo-controlled	24	phase 3	Completed/ failed	NCT00414440	[131]
6	Tolvaptan	V2-receptor antagonist	parallel-arm, double blind and placebo controlled	36	phase 3	Completed	NCT00428948	[123]

Table 1. (Continued)

	Drugs	Signaling pathway	Study design	Treatment duration (months)	Clinical phase trial	Clinical trial status	Clinical trials Gov. identifier	Ref.
7	Lisinopril and Telmisartan (HALT PKD)1	ACE inhibitor [lisinopril] and angiotensin II receptor blocker (ARB) [telmisartan]	Randomized, double-blind and placebo controlled	72	phase 3	Ongoing	NCT00283686	[144, 145]
8	Pravastatin1	A (HMG coA) reductase inhibitors	Randomized, doubleblind, placebo-controlled	36	phase 3	Ongoing	NCT00456365	[146, 147]
9	Somatostatin	cAMP inhibitor pathway in ADKPD and ADPLD	Randomized, single-blind and placebo controlled	36	phase 3	Ongoing	NCT00309283	not available
10	Bosutinib	c-Src inhibitor	Randomized, double-blind and placebo controlled	24	phase 2	Ongoing	NCT01233869	[148]
12	Triptolide	Restore intracellular Ca2+ signaling and inhibit cell proliferation	Randomized and open-label	36	phase 2	Ongoing	NCT00801268	[149-151]

Conclusion

Since the discovery of *PKD1* and *PKD2*, there has been tremendous progress in studying disease pathophysiology. As a result, many promising drugs have been and are being developed to slow halt or reverse the progression of cystic disease. Given the complexity of disease and the important extrarenal features, it is likely that a range of specific drugs will be needed to treat patients with ADPKD.

References

[1]   P. D. Wilson, Polycystic kidney disease. *The New England journal of medicine* 350, 151 (Jan 8, 2004).

[2]   W. E. Braun, Autosomal dominant polycystic kidney disease: emerging concepts of pathogenesis and new treatments. *Cleve Clin. J. Med.* 76, 97 (Feb, 2009).

[3]   US Renal Data System: USRDS 2008 Annual Data Report. *The National Institutes of Health, National Institute of Diabetes and Digestive and Kidney Disease* Bethesda, MD, (2008).

[4]   Polycystic kidney disease: the complete structure of the PKD1 gene and its protein. The International Polycystic Kidney Disease Consortium. *Cell* 81, 289 (Apr 21, 1995).

[5]   The polycystic kidney disease 1 gene encodes a 14 kb transcript and lies within a duplicated region on chromosome 16. The European Polycystic Kidney Disease Consortium. *Cell* 77, 881 (Jun 17, 1994).

[6]   T. Mochizuki *et al.*, PKD2, a gene for polycystic kidney disease that encodes an integral membrane protein. *Science* 272, 1339 (May 31, 1996).

[7]   C. J. Ward *et al.*, The gene mutated in autosomal recessive polycystic kidney disease encodes a large, receptor-like protein. *Nature genetics* 30, 259 (Mar, 2002).

[8]   V. E. Torres, P. C. Harris, Polycystic kidney disease in 2011: Connecting the dots toward a polycystic kidney disease therapy. *Nature reviews. Nephrology* 8, 66 (Feb, 2012).

[9]   P. C. Harris, V. E. Torres, in *GeneReviews,* R. A. Pagon, T. D. Bird, C. R. Dolan, K. Stephens, M. P. Adam, Eds. (Seattle (WA), 1993).

[10] P. C. Harris, V. E. Torres, Polycystic kidney disease. *Annual review of medicine* 60, 321 (2009).

[11] S. M. Nauli *et al.*, Loss of polycystin-1 in human cyst-lining epithelia leads to ciliary dysfunction. *Journal of the American Society of Nephrology : JASN* 17, 1015 (Apr, 2006).

[12] S. M. Nauli *et al.*, Polycystins 1 and 2 mediate mechanosensation in the primary cilium of kidney cells. *Nature genetics* 33, 129 (Feb, 2003).

[13] B. K. Yoder, X. Hou, L. M. Guay-Woodford, The polycystic kidney disease proteins, polycystin-1, polycystin-2, polaris, and cystin, are co-localized in renal cilia. *Journal of the American Society of Nephrology : JASN* 13, 2508 (Oct, 2002).

[14] R. Sandford *et al.*, Comparative analysis of the polycystic kidney disease 1 (PKD1) gene reveals an integral membrane glycoprotein with multiple evolutionary conserved domains. *Human molecular genetics* 6, 1483 (Sep, 1997).

[15] J. Hughes *et al.*, The polycystic kidney disease 1 (PKD1) gene encodes a novel protein with multiple cell recognition domains. *Nature genetics* 10, 151 (Jun, 1995).

[16] J. Van Adelsberg, S. Chamberlain, V. D'Agati, Polycystin expression is temporally and spatially regulated during renal development. *The American journal of physiology* 272, F602 (May, 1997).

[17] L. Geng *et al.*, Distribution and developmentally regulated expression of murine polycystin. *The American journal of physiology* 272, F451 (Apr, 1997).

[18] S. Gonzalez-Perrett *et al.*, Polycystin-2, the protein mutated in autosomal dominant polycystic kidney disease (ADPKD), is a Ca2+-permeable nonselective cation channel. *Proceedings of the National Academy of Sciences of the United States of America* 98, 1182 (Jan 30, 2001).

[19] P. Koulen *et al.*, Polycystin-2 is an intracellular calcium release channel. *Nature cell biology* 4, 191 (Mar, 2002).

[20] B. S. Muntean, S. Jin, S. M. Nauli, Primary Cilia are Mechanosensory Organelles with Chemosensory Roles. *Mechanical Stretch and Cytokines, Mechanosensitivity in Cells and Tissues* 5, 201 (2012).

[21] N. B. Gilula, P. Satir, The ciliary necklace. A ciliary membrane specialization. *The Journal of cell biology* 53, 494 (May, 1972).

[22] A. Molla-Herman *et al.*, The ciliary pocket: an endocytic membrane domain at the base of primary and motile cilia. *Journal of cell science* 123, 1785 (May 15, 2010).

[23] H. L. Kee *et al.*, A size-exclusion permeability barrier and nucleoporins characterize a ciliary pore complex that regulates transport into cilia. *Nature cell biology* 14, 431 (Apr, 2012).

[24] R. Rohatgi, W. J. Snell, The ciliary membrane. *Current opinion in cell biology* 22, 541 (Aug, 2010).

[25] S. Wang *et al.*, Fibrocystin/polyductin, found in the same protein complex with polycystin-2, regulates calcium responses in kidney epithelia. *Molecular and cellular biology* 27, 3241 (Apr, 2007).

[26] C. Xu *et al.*, Human ADPKD primary cyst epithelial cells with a novel, single codon deletion in the PKD1 gene exhibit defective ciliary polycystin localization and loss of flow-induced Ca2+ signaling. *American journal of physiology. Renal physiology* 292, F930 (Mar, 2007).

[27] S. H. Low *et al.*, Polycystin-1, STAT6, and P100 function in a pathway that transduces ciliary mechanosensation and is activated in polycystic kidney disease. *Developmental cell* 10, 57 (Jan, 2006).

[28] V. Chauvet *et al.*, Mechanical stimuli induce cleavage and nuclear translocation of the polycystin-1 C terminus. *The Journal of clinical investigation* 114, 1433 (Nov, 2004).

[29] E. Fischer *et al.*, Defective planar cell polarity in polycystic kidney disease. *Nature genetics* 38, 21 (Jan, 2006).

[30] V. Patel *et al.*, Acute kidney injury and aberrant planar cell polarity induce cyst formation in mice lacking renal cilia. *Human molecular genetics* 17, 1578 (Jun 1, 2008).

[31] W. A. AbouAlaiwi, S. Ratnam, R. L. Booth, J. V. Shah, S. M. Nauli, Endothelial cells from humans and mice with polycystic kidney disease are characterized by polyploidy and chromosome segregation defects through survivin down-regulation. *Human molecular genetics* 20, 354 (Jan 15, 2011).

[32] A. Masoumi, B. Reed-Gitomer, C. Kelleher, M. R. Bekheirnia, R. W. Schrier, Developments in the management of autosomal dominant polycystic kidney disease. *Therapeutics and clinical risk management* 4, 393 (Apr, 2008).

[33] K. T. Bae *et al.*, Magnetic resonance imaging evaluation of hepatic cysts in early autosomal-dominant polycystic kidney disease: the Consortium for Radiologic Imaging Studies of Polycystic Kidney Disease cohort. *Clinical journal of the American Society of Nephrology : CJASN* 1, 64 (Jan, 2006).

[34]   V. E. Torres, P. C. Harris, Y. Pirson, Autosomal dominant polycystic kidney disease. *Lancet* 369, 1287 (Apr 14, 2007).

[35]   S. Abdul-Majeed, S. M. Nauli, Polycystic diseases in visceral organs. *Obstetrics and gynecology international* 2011, 609370 (2011).

[36]   J. H. Grendell, T. H. Ermak, Anatomy, histology, embryology, and developmental anomalies of the pancreas. *Sleisenger and Fordtran's Gastrointestinal and Liver Disease*, 761 (1998).

[37]   O. Basar *et al.*, Recurrent pancreatitis in a patient with autosomal-dominant polycystic kidney disease. *Pancreatology* 6, 160 (2006).

[38]   R. Torra *et al.*, Ultrasonographic study of pancreatic cysts in autosomal dominant polycystic kidney disease. *Clinical nephrology* 47, 19 (Jan, 1997).

[39]   D. A. Cano, N. S. Murcia, G. J. Pazour, M. Hebrok, Orpk mouse model of polycystic kidney disease reveals essential role of primary cilia in pancreatic tissue organization. *Development* 131, 3457 (Jul, 2004).

[40]   J. H. Moyer *et al.*, Candidate gene associated with a mutation causing recessive polycystic kidney disease in mice. *Science* 264, 1329 (May 27, 1994).

[41]   D. A. Cano, S. Sekine, M. Hebrok, Primary cilia deletion in pancreatic epithelial cells results in cyst formation and pancreatitis. *Gastroenterology* 131, 1856 (Dec, 2006).

[42]   S. Y. Li *et al.*, Recurrent retroperitoneal abscess due to perforated colonic diverticulitis in a patient with polycystic kidney disease. *Journal of the Chinese Medical Association : JCMA* 72, 153 (Mar, 2009).

[43]   E. D. Lederman, G. McCoy, D. J. Conti, E. C. Lee, Diverticulitis and polycystic kidney disease. *The American surgeon* 66, 200 (Feb, 2000).

[44]   E. D. Lederman, D. J. Conti, N. Lempert, T. P. Singh, E. C. Lee, Complicated diverticulitis following renal transplantation. *Diseases of the colon and rectum* 41, 613 (May, 1998).

[45]   Z. H. Bajwa, K. A. Sial, A. B. Malik, T. I. Steinman, Pain patterns in patients with polycystic kidney disease. *Kidney international* 66, 1561 (Oct, 2004).

[46]   T. Ecder, R. W. Schrier, Cardiovascular abnormalities in autosomal-dominant polycystic kidney disease. *Nature reviews. Nephrology* 5, 221 (Apr, 2009).

[47]   G. M. Fick, A. M. Johnson, W. S. Hammond, P. A. Gabow, Causes of death in autosomal dominant polycystic kidney disease. *Journal of the American Society of Nephrology : JASN* 5, 2048 (Jun, 1995).

[48] A. B. Chapman, R. W. Schrier, Pathogenesis of hypertension in autosomal dominant polycystic kidney disease. *Seminars in nephrology* 11, 653 (Nov, 1991).

[49] A. B. Chapman, K. Stepniakowski, F. Rahbari-Oskoui, Hypertension in autosomal dominant polycystic kidney disease. *Advances in chronic kidney disease* 17, 153 (Mar, 2010).

[50] C. L. Kelleher, K. K. McFann, A. M. Johnson, R. W. Schrier, Characteristics of hypertension in young adults with autosomal dominant polycystic kidney disease compared with the general U.S. population. *American journal of hypertension* 17, 1029 (Nov, 2004).

[51] R. W. Schrier, A. M. Johnson, K. McFann, A. B. Chapman, The role of parental hypertension in the frequency and age of diagnosis of hypertension in offspring with autosomal-dominant polycystic kidney disease. *Kidney international* 64, 1792 (Nov, 2003).

[52] S. M. Nauli, X. Jin, B. P. Hierck, The mechanosensory role of primary cilia in vascular hypertension. *International journal of vascular medicine* 2011, 376281 (2011).

[53] M. Y. Chang, A. C. Ong, Endothelin in polycystic kidney disease. *Contributions to nephrology* 172, 200 (2011).

[54] Y. Kawanabe *et al.*, Cilostazol prevents endothelin-induced smooth muscle constriction and proliferation. *PloS one* 7, e44476 (2012).

[55] Y. Kawanabe, S. M. Nauli, Endothelin. *Cellular and molecular life sciences : CMLS* 68, 195 (Jan, 2011).

[56] A. C. Ong *et al.*, An endothelin-1 mediated autocrine growth loop involved in human renal tubular regeneration. *Kidney international* 48, 390 (Aug, 1995).

[57] A. C. Ong *et al.*, Human tubular-derived endothelin in the paracrine regulation of renal interstitial fibroblast function. *Experimental nephrology* 2, 134 (Mar-Apr, 1994).

[58] M. Y. Chang *et al.*, Haploinsufficiency of Pkd2 is associated with increased tubular cell proliferation and interstitial fibrosis in two murine Pkd2 models. *Nephrology, dialysis, transplantation : official publication of the European Dialysis and Transplant Association - European Renal Association* 21, 2078 (Aug, 2006).

[59] B. Hocher *et al.*, Renal endothelin system in polycystic kidney disease. *Journal of the American Society of Nephrology : JASN* 9, 1169 (Jul, 1998).

[60] C. Munemura, J. Uemasu, H. Kawasaki, Epidermal growth factor and endothelin in cyst fluid from autosomal dominant polycystic kidney

disease cases: possible evidence of heterogeneity in cystogenesis. *American journal of kidney diseases : the official journal of the National Kidney Foundation* 24, 561 (Oct, 1994).

[61] R. Giusti *et al.*, Plasma concentration of endothelin and arterial pressure in patients with ADPKD. *Contributions to nephrology* 115, 118 (1995).

[62] D. Wang, J. Iversen, S. Strandgaard, Endothelium-dependent relaxation of small resistance vessels is impaired in patients with autosomal dominant polycystic kidney disease. *Journal of the American Society of Nephrology : JASN* 11, 1371 (Aug, 2000).

[63] M. A. Al-Nimri *et al.*, Endothelial-derived vasoactive mediators in polycystic kidney disease. *Kidney international* 63, 1776 (May, 2003).

[64] Y. Ge, P. K. Stricklett, A. K. Hughes, M. Yanagisawa, D. E. Kohan, Collecting duct-specific knockout of the endothelin A receptor alters renal vasopressin responsiveness, but not sodium excretion or blood pressure. *American journal of physiology. Renal physiology* 289, F692 (Oct, 2005).

[65] Y. Ge *et al.*, Collecting duct-specific knockout of endothelin-1 alters vasopressin regulation of urine osmolality. *American journal of physiology. Renal physiology* 288, F912 (May, 2005).

[66] D. E. Kohan, The renal medullary endothelin system in control of sodium and water excretion and systemic blood pressure. *Current opinion in nephrology and hypertension* 15, 34 (Jan, 2006).

[67] V. E. Torres, P. C. Harris, Autosomal dominant polycystic kidney disease: the last 3 years. *Kidney international* 76, 149 (Jul, 2009).

[68] M. Y. Chang, E. Parker, M. El Nahas, J. L. Haylor, A. C. Ong, Endothelin B receptor blockade accelerates disease progression in a murine model of autosomal dominant polycystic kidney disease. *Journal of the American Society of Nephrology : JASN* 18, 560 (Feb, 2007).

[69] R. W. Schrier, Renal volume, renin-angiotensin-aldosterone system, hypertension, and left ventricular hypertrophy in patients with autosomal dominant polycystic kidney disease. *Journal of the American Society of Nephrology : JASN* 20, 1888 (Sep, 2009).

[70] S. Abdul-Majeed, S. M. Nauli, Dopamine receptor type 5 in the primary cilia has dual chemo- and mechano-sensory roles. *Hypertension* 58, 325 (Aug, 2011).

[71] S. Abdul-Majeed, B. C. Moloney, S. M. Nauli, Mechanisms regulating cilia growth and cilia function in endothelial cells. *Cellular and molecular life sciences : CMLS* 69, 165 (Jan, 2012).

[72] W. A. AbouAlaiwi *et al.*, Ciliary polycystin-2 is a mechanosensitive calcium channel involved in nitric oxide signaling cascades. *Circulation research* 104, 860 (Apr 10, 2009).

[73] S. M. Nauli *et al.*, Endothelial cilia are fluid shear sensors that regulate calcium signaling and nitric oxide production through polycystin-1. *Circulation* 117, 1161 (Mar 4, 2008).

[74] A. C. Ong *et al.*, Coordinate expression of the autosomal dominant polycystic kidney disease proteins, polycystin-2 and polycystin-1, in normal and cystic tissue. *The American journal of pathology* 154, 1721 (Jun, 1999).

[75] S. Abdul-Majeed, S. M. Nauli, Calcium-mediated mechanisms of cystic expansion. *Biochimica et biophysica acta* 1812, 1281 (Oct, 2011).

[76] N. Hateboer *et al.*, Location of mutations within the PKD2 gene influences clinical outcome. *Kidney international* 57, 1444 (Apr, 2000).

[77] N. Hateboer *et al.*, Comparison of phenotypes of polycystic kidney disease types 1 and 2. European PKD1-PKD2 Study Group. *Lancet* 353, 103 (Jan 9, 1999).

[78] S. Hassane *et al.*, Pathogenic sequence for dissecting aneurysm formation in a hypomorphic polycystic kidney disease 1 mouse model. *Arteriosclerosis, thrombosis, and vascular biology* 27, 2177 (Oct, 2007).

[79] Z. L. Brookes *et al.*, Pkd2 mesenteric vessels exhibit a primary defect in endothelium-dependent vasodilatation restored by rosiglitazone. *American journal of physiology. Heart and circulatory physiology* 304, H33 (Jan 1, 2013).

[80] P. A. Gabow *et al.*, Renal structure and hypertension in autosomal dominant polycystic kidney disease. *Kidney international* 38, 1177 (Dec, 1990).

[81] M. Loghman-Adham, C. E. Soto, T. Inagami, L. Cassis, The intrarenal renin-angiotensin system in autosomal dominant polycystic kidney disease. *American journal of physiology. Renal physiology* 287, F775 (Oct, 2004).

[82] A. B. Chapman, P. A. Gabow, Hypertension in autosomal dominant polycystic kidney disease. *Kidney international. Supplement* 61, S71 (Oct, 1997).

[83] E. A. McPherson *et al.*, Chymase-like angiotensin II-generating activity in end-stage human autosomal dominant polycystic kidney disease. *Journal of the American Society of Nephrology : JASN* 15, 493 (Feb, 2004).

[84] P. J. Azurmendi *et al.*, Early renal and vascular changes in ADPKD patients with low-grade albumin excretion and normal renal function. *Nephrology, dialysis, transplantation : official publication of the European Dialysis and Transplant Association - European Renal Association* 24, 2458 (Aug, 2009).

[85] C. T. Itty, A. Farshid, G. Talaulikar, Spontaneous coronary artery dissection in a woman with polycystic kidney disease. *American journal of kidney diseases : the official journal of the National Kidney Foundation* 53, 518 (Mar, 2009).

[86] C. Boulter *et al.*, Cardiovascular, skeletal, and renal defects in mice with a targeted disruption of the Pkd1 gene. *Proceedings of the National Academy of Sciences of the United States of America* 98, 12174 (Oct 9, 2001).

[87] M. A. Arnaout, Molecular genetics and pathogenesis of autosomal dominant polycystic kidney disease. *Annual review of medicine* 52, 93 (2001).

[88] J. Neumann, G. Ligtenberg, I. H. Klein, P. J. Blankestijn, Pathogenesis and treatment of hypertension in polycystic kidney disease. *Current opinion in nephrology and hypertension* 11, 517 (Sep, 2002).

[89] I. H. Klein, G. Ligtenberg, P. L. Oey, H. A. Koomans, P. J. Blankestijn, Sympathetic activity is increased in polycystic kidney disease and is associated with hypertension. *Journal of the American Society of Nephrology : JASN* 12, 2427 (Nov, 2001).

[90] R. Zeltner, R. Poliak, B. Stiasny, R. E. Schmieder, B. D. Schulze, Renal and cardiac effects of antihypertensive treatment with ramipril vs metoprolol in autosomal dominant polycystic kidney disease. *Nephrology, dialysis, transplantation : official publication of the European Dialysis and Transplant Association - European Renal Association* 23, 573 (Feb, 2008).

[91] M. J. Koren, R. B. Devereux, P. N. Casale, D. D. Savage, J. H. Laragh, Relation of left ventricular mass and geometry to morbidity and mortality in uncomplicated essential hypertension. *Annals of internal medicine* 114, 345 (Mar 1, 1991).

[92] P. A. Gabow *et al.*, Factors affecting the progression of renal disease in autosomal-dominant polycystic kidney disease. *Kidney international* 41, 1311 (May, 1992).

[93] A. B. Chapman *et al.*, Left ventricular hypertrophy in autosomal dominant polycystic kidney disease. *Journal of the American Society of Nephrology : JASN* 8, 1292 (Aug, 1997).

[94] M. A. Cadnapaphornchai, K. McFann, J. D. Strain, A. Masoumi, R. W. Schrier, Increased left ventricular mass in children with autosomal dominant polycystic kidney disease and borderline hypertension. *Kidney international* 74, 1192 (Nov, 2008).

[95] A. Bardaji *et al.*, Cardiac involvement in autosomal-dominant polycystic kidney disease: a hypertensive heart disease. *Clinical nephrology* 56, 211 (Sep, 2001).

[96] H. Oflaz *et al.*, Biventricular diastolic dysfunction in patients with autosomal-dominant polycystic kidney disease. *Kidney international* 68, 2244 (Nov, 2005).

[97] P. Verdecchia *et al.*, Circadian blood pressure changes and left ventricular hypertrophy in essential hypertension. *Circulation* 81, 528 (Feb, 1990).

[98] T. C. Li Kam Wa, A. M. Macnicol, M. L. Watson, Ambulatory blood pressure in hypertensive patients with autosomal dominant polycystic kidney disease. *Nephrology, dialysis, transplantation : official publication of the European Dialysis and Transplant Association - European Renal Association* 12, 2075 (Oct, 1997).

[99] F. A. Valero *et al.*, Ambulatory blood pressure and left ventricular mass in normotensive patients with autosomal dominant polycystic kidney disease. *Journal of the American Society of Nephrology : JASN* 10, 1020 (May, 1999).

[100] A. Lumiaho *et al.*, Insulin resistance is related to left ventricular hypertrophy in patients with polycystic kidney disease type 1. *American journal of kidney diseases : the official journal of the National Kidney Foundation* 41, 1219 (Jun, 2003).

[101] G. Lembo *et al.*, Abnormal sympathetic overactivity evoked by insulin in the skeletal muscle of patients with essential hypertension. *The Journal of clinical investigation* 90, 24 (Jul, 1992).

[102] T. Ecder, R. W. Schrier, Hypertension and left ventricular hypertrophy in autosomal dominant polycystic kidney disease. *Expert review of cardiovascular therapy* 2, 369 (May, 2004).

[103] P. M. Ruggieri *et al.*, Occult intracranial aneurysms in polycystic kidney disease: screening with MR angiography. *Radiology* 191, 33 (Apr, 1994).

[104] A. P. Rocchini, C. Moorehead, S. DeRemer, T. L. Goodfriend, D. L. Ball, Hyperinsulinemia and the aldosterone and pressor responses to angiotensin II. *Hypertension* 15, 861 (Jun, 1990).

[105] S. Graf *et al.*, Intracranial aneurysms and dolichoectasia in autosomal dominant polycystic kidney disease. *Nephrology, dialysis, transplantation : official publication of the European Dialysis and Transplant Association - European Renal Association* 17, 819 (May, 2002).

[106] M. M. Belz *et al.*, Recurrence of intracranial aneurysms in autosomal-dominant polycystic kidney disease. *Kidney international* 63, 1824 (May, 2003).

[107] M. M. Belz *et al.*, Familial clustering of ruptured intracranial aneurysms in autosomal dominant polycystic kidney disease. *American journal of kidney diseases : the official journal of the National Kidney Foundation* 38, 770 (Oct, 2001).

[108] H. Hadimeri, C. Lamm, G. Nyberg, Coronary aneurysms in patients with autosomal dominant polycystic kidney disease. *Journal of the American Society of Nephrology : JASN* 9, 837 (May, 1998).

[109] R. Torra *et al.*, Abdominal aortic aneurysms and autosomal dominant polycystic kidney disease. *Journal of the American Society of Nephrology : JASN* 7, 2483 (Nov, 1996).

[110] T. Ecder *et al.*, Reversal of left ventricular hypertrophy with angiotensin converting enzyme inhibition in hypertensive patients with autosomal dominant polycystic kidney disease. *Nephrology, dialysis, transplantation : official publication of the European Dialysis and Transplant Association - European Renal Association* 14, 1113 (May, 1999).

[111] M. Y. Chang, A. C. Ong, Mechanism-based therapeutics for autosomal dominant polycystic kidney disease: recent progress and future prospects. *Nephron. Clinical practice* 120, c25 (2012).

[112] M. Y. Chang, A. C. Ong, New treatments for autosomal dominant polycystic kidney disease. *British journal of clinical pharmacology*, (Apr 18, 2013).

[113] G. Aguiari, L. Catizone, L. Del Senno, Multidrug therapy for polycystic kidney disease: a review and perspective. *American journal of nephrology* 37, 175 (2013).

[114] T. Yamaguchi, G. A. Reif, J. P. Calvet, D. P. Wallace, Sorafenib inhibits cAMP-dependent ERK activation, cell proliferation, and in vitro cyst growth of human ADPKD cyst epithelial cells. *American journal of physiology. Renal physiology* 299, F944 (Nov, 2010).

[115] A. J. Streets, O. Wessely, D. J. Peters, A. C. Ong, Hyperphosphorylation of polycystin-2 at a critical residue in disease reveals an essential role for

polycystin-1-regulated dephosphorylation. *Human molecular genetics* 22, 1924 (May 15, 2013).

[116] S. Terryn, A. Ho, R. Beauwens, O. Devuyst, Fluid transport and cystogenesis in autosomal dominant polycystic kidney disease. *Biochimica et biophysica acta* 1812, 1314 (Oct, 2011).

[117] S. Nagao *et al.*, Increased water intake decreases progression of polycystic kidney disease in the PCK rat. *Journal of the American Society of Nephrology : JASN* 17, 2220 (Aug, 2006).

[118] X. Wang, Y. Wu, C. J. Ward, P. C. Harris, V. E. Torres, Vasopressin directly regulates cyst growth in polycystic kidney disease. *Journal of the American Society of Nephrology : JASN* 19, 102 (Jan, 2008).

[119] V. H. Gattone, 2nd, X. Wang, P. C. Harris, V. E. Torres, Inhibition of renal cystic disease development and progression by a vasopressin V2 receptor antagonist. *Nature medicine* 9, 1323 (Oct, 2003).

[120] V. E. Torres *et al.*, Effective treatment of an orthologous model of autosomal dominant polycystic kidney disease. *Nature medicine* 10, 363 (Apr, 2004).

[121] V. H. Gattone, 2nd, R. L. Maser, C. Tian, J. M. Rosenberg, M. G. Branden, Developmental expression of urine concentration-associated genes and their altered expression in murine infantile-type polycystic kidney disease. *Developmental genetics* 24, 309 (1999).

[122] X. Wang, V. Gattone, 2nd, P. C. Harris, V. E. Torres, Effectiveness of vasopressin V2 receptor antagonists OPC-31260 and OPC-41061 on polycystic kidney disease development in the PCK rat. *Journal of the American Society of Nephrology : JASN* 16, 846 (Apr, 2005).

[123] V. E. Torres *et al.*, Tolvaptan in patients with autosomal dominant polycystic kidney disease. *The New England journal of medicine* 367, 2407 (Dec 20, 2012).

[124] C. Boehlke *et al.*, Primary cilia regulate mTORC1 activity and cell size through Lkb1. *Nature cell biology* 12, 1115 (Nov, 2010).

[125] O. Ibraghimov-Beskrovnaya, T. A. Natoli, mTOR signaling in polycystic kidney disease. *Trends in molecular medicine* 17, 625 (Nov, 2011).

[126] C. S. Bonnet *et al.*, Defects in cell polarity underlie TSC and ADPKD-associated cystogenesis. *Human molecular genetics* 18, 2166 (Jun 15, 2009).

[127] J. Huang, C. C. Dibble, M. Matsuzaki, B. D. Manning, The TSC1-TSC2 complex is required for proper activation of mTOR complex 2. *Molecular and cellular biology* 28, 4104 (Jun, 2008).

[128] J. M. Shillingford *et al.*, The mTOR pathway is regulated by polycystin-1, and its inhibition reverses renal cystogenesis in polycystic kidney disease. *Proceedings of the National Academy of Sciences of the United States of America* 103, 5466 (Apr 4, 2006).

[129] M. Wu *et al.*, Everolimus retards cyst growth and preserves kidney function in a rodent model for polycystic kidney disease. *Kidney and blood pressure research* 30, 253 (2007).

[130] P. R. Wahl *et al.*, Inhibition of mTOR with sirolimus slows disease progression in Han:SPRD rats with autosomal dominant polycystic kidney disease (ADPKD). *Nephrology, dialysis, transplantation : official publication of the European Dialysis and Transplant Association - European Renal Association* 21, 598 (Mar, 2006).

[131] G. Walz *et al.*, Everolimus in patients with autosomal dominant polycystic kidney disease. *The New England journal of medicine* 363, 830 (Aug 26, 2010).

[132] A. L. Serra *et al.*, Sirolimus and kidney growth in autosomal dominant polycystic kidney disease. *The New England journal of medicine* 363, 820 (Aug 26, 2010).

[133] N. N. Zheleznova, P. D. Wilson, A. Staruschenko, Epidermal growth factor-mediated proliferation and sodium transport in normal and PKD epithelial cells. *Biochimica et biophysica acta* 1812, 1301 (Oct, 2011).

[134] F. Zeng, A. B. Singh, R. C. Harris, The role of the EGF family of ligands and receptors in renal development, physiology and pathophysiology. *Experimental cell research* 315, 602 (Feb 15, 2009).

[135] F. Zeng, M. Z. Zhang, A. B. Singh, R. Zent, R. C. Harris, ErbB4 isoforms selectively regulate growth factor induced Madin-Darby canine kidney cell tubulogenesis. *Molecular biology of the cell* 18, 4446 (Nov, 2007).

[136] J. Du, P. D. Wilson, Abnormal polarization of EGF receptors and autocrine stimulation of cyst epithelial growth in human ADPKD. *The American journal of physiology* 269, C487 (Aug, 1995).

[137] P. D. Wilson, J. Du, J. T. Norman, Autocrine, endocrine and paracrine regulation of growth abnormalities in autosomal dominant polycystic kidney disease. *European journal of cell biology* 61, 131 (Jun, 1993).

[138] V. E. Torres *et al.*, EGF receptor tyrosine kinase inhibition attenuates the development of PKD in Han:SPRD rats. *Kidney international* 64, 1573 (Nov, 2003).

[139] G. Aguiari *et al.*, Polycystin-1 regulates amphiregulin expression through CREB and AP1 signalling: implications in ADPKD cell proliferation. *J. Mol. Med. (Berl)* 90, 1267 (Nov, 2012).

[140] M. C. Hogan *et al.*, Randomized clinical trial of long-acting somatostatin for autosomal dominant polycystic kidney and liver disease. *Journal of the American Society of Nephrology : JASN* 21, 1052 (Jun, 2010).

[141] T. V. Masyuk, A. I. Masyuk, V. E. Torres, P. C. Harris, N. F. Larusso, Octreotide inhibits hepatic cystogenesis in a rodent model of polycystic liver disease by reducing cholangiocyte adenosine 3',5'-cyclic monophosphate. *Gastroenterology* 132, 1104 (Mar, 2007).

[142] L. van Keimpema *et al.*, Lanreotide reduces the volume of polycystic liver: a randomized, double-blind, placebo-controlled trial. *Gastroenterology* 137, 1661 (Nov, 2009).

[143] N. Perico *et al.*, Sirolimus therapy to halt the progression of ADPKD. *Journal of the American Society of Nephrology : JASN* 21, 1031 (Jun, 2010).

[144] V. E. Torres *et al.*, Analysis of baseline parameters in the HALT polycystic kidney disease trials. *Kidney international* 81, 577 (Mar, 2012).

[145] A. M. Sengul, Y. Altuntas, A. Kurklu, L. Aydin, Beneficial effect of lisinopril plus telmisartan in patients with type 2 diabetes, microalbuminuria and hypertension. *Diabetes research and clinical practice* 71, 210 (Feb, 2006).

[146] M. A. Cadnapaphornchai *et al.*, Effect of statin therapy on disease progression in pediatric ADPKD: design and baseline characteristics of participants. *Contemporary clinical trials* 32, 437 (May, 2011).

[147] R. W. Schrier, Optimal care of autosomal dominant polycystic kidney disease patients. *Nephrology (Carlton)* 11, 124 (Apr, 2006).

[148] J. Elliott, N. N. Zheleznova, P. D. Wilson, c-Src inactivation reduces renal epithelial cell-matrix adhesion, proliferation, and cyst formation. *American journal of physiology. Cell physiology* 301, C522 (Aug, 2011).

[149] S. J. Leuenroth, N. Bencivenga, H. Chahboune, F. Hyder, C. M. Crews, Triptolide reduces cyst formation in a neonatal to adult transition Pkd1 model of ADPKD. *Nephrology, dialysis, transplantation : official publication of the European Dialysis and Transplant Association - European Renal Association* 25, 2187 (Jul, 2010).

[150] S. J. Leuenroth, N. Bencivenga, P. Igarashi, S. Somlo, C. M. Crews, Triptolide reduces cystogenesis in a model of ADPKD. *Journal of the American Society of Nephrology : JASN* 19, 1659 (Sep, 2008).

[151] S. J. Leuenroth *et al.*, Triptolide is a traditional Chinese medicine-derived inhibitor of polycystic kidney disease. *Proceedings of the National Academy of Sciences of the United States of America* 104, 4389 (Mar 13, 2007).

[152] R. J. Kolb, S. M. Nauli, Ciliary dysfunction in polycystic kidney disease: an emerging model with polarizing potential. *Frontiers in bioscience : a journal and virtual library* 13, 4451 (2008).

[153] W. A. Abou Alaiwi, S. T. Lo, S. M. Nauli, Primary cilia: highly sophisticated biological sensors. *Sensors (Basel)* 9, 7003 (2009).

[154] S. Ratnam, S. M. Nauli, Hypertension in Autosomal Dominant Polycystic Kidney Disease: A Clinical and Basic Science Perspective. *Int. J. Nephrol Urol.* 2, 294 (2010).

In: Autosomal Dominant Disorders   ISBN: 978-1-62808-760-4
Editors: P. Marciano and D. M. Lanza © 2013 Nova Science Publishers, Inc.

Chapter 2

Hereditary Haemorrhagic Telangiectasia or Rendu-Osler-Weber Syndrome

Roberto Zarrabeitia[2], Cristina Amado[2],
Virginia Albiñana[1] and Luisa-María Botella[1]
[1]Center for Biological Investigations (CIB) , Spanish Research Council,
(CSIC). Madrid. CIBERER
[2]Sierrallana Hospital, Reference Hospital for HHT in Spain, Torrelavega,
Santander, Spain. IFIMAV

Abstract

Hereditary Haemorrhagic Telangiectasia (HHT) or Rendu Osler Weber syndrome (OMIM 187300/ORPHA774) is a vascular hereditary autosomic dominant multiorganic dysplasia,. Prevalence is in between 1 to 5,000/8,000 inhabitants around 65,000 in Europe, and 200,000 in USA); although due to founder effect, and insulation, it is higher in some regions as the Jura in France, Funen Island in Denmark and Caribbean Dutch Antilles where the prevalence may be 1 in 1,200 inhabitants. Diagnosis is based on the clinical criteria of Curaçao (Shovlin et al., 2000): epistaxis, telangiectases, first degree relative with HHT, and visceral arteriovenous malformations (AVMs), mainly in lung, liver and brain. For a positive diagnosis, 3 out of the 4 previous criteria are required. A positive genetic test implies also a positive diagnosis.

The clinical diagnosis requires then a detailed medical screening, with involvement of different medical specialities. Penetrance of the disease is variable increasing with age.

Pulmonary arteriovenous malformations (PAVMs) occur in aproximately 50% of patients, hepatic involvement in up to 70%, brain AVMs in 10% and spinal in 1%. However the most frequent clinical manifestation of HHT is epistaxis (nose bleeding) normally from light to moderate that affects 93% of patients and is present before the age of 21 in 90 % of cases (Faughnan et al., 2009).

The genetic origin of the disease is due to mutations of genes involved in the TGB-β pathway, critical for the normal development of blood vessels (Fernández et al. 2006). The first gene identified was *Endoglin (ENG)*, responsible for the 39-59% of the HHT cases (HHT 1); shortly after, *ALK1/(ACVRL1)* was discovered to be involved in 25-57% of cases (HHT2). In around 2% of the HHT patients, the mutation is located in the *MADH4/Smad4* gene leading to a combined syndrome of Juvenile Polyposis and HHT (JPHT). A third and a fourth locus have been mapped on chromosomes 5 and 7 with no genes identified at the moment. Endoglin plays a key role in vasculogenesis and arterial/venous differentiation in embryos, as well as in angiogenesis and neovascularization processes in the adult; ALK1 is responsible for the events occurring during the activation phase of angiogenesis. Haploinsufficiency is accepted as the mechanism of pathogenicity for the HHT.

Introduction

Hereditary Haemorrhagic Telangiectasia (HHT) or Rendu Osler Weber syndrome (OMIM 187300/CIE9 448.0/ORPHA774) is a genetic disease with dominant inheritance pattern leading to a vascular dysplasia characterized by the presence of lesions ranging from small vessel enlargements (telangiectases) to complex arteriovenous malformations (AVMs) or shunts that can potentially affect any organ but mainly lungs, brain, liver and gastrointestinal tract. First described [1] by Henry Gawen Sutton in 1864, it was Henry Rendu in 1886 who recognized it as a different entity from the haemophilia [2]. William Bart Osler in 1901 and Frederick Parks Weber in 1907 published the first series of cases [3,4] but it was in 1909, when Hanes introduced the actual terminology of HHT [5]. Microscopical anatomical findings rely on the presence in a capillary vessel of a direct communication bettween artery and vein with absence of the intermedium capillary net [6,7]. In the initial phase of the development of the telangiectasia, a dilatation of the postcapilary venules in the horizontal upper plexus in the papillary dermis occurs with the presence of a perivascular infiltration of lymphocytes, monocytes and macrophages; in the intermediate phase, when the lession reachs a diameter of 0.5 mm, the walls of the postcapillary venule enlarge due to the increase in the number of perycites while the arteriole can be dilated but still connected by a short capillary system with the venule; at the end when the telangiectasia is completely formed (2 mm), the venules are markedly dilated, elongated and twisted occupying the whole dermis. These venules have between 8 and 11 layers of plain muscle and disperse quantities of collagen with no elastic fibers; direct connection between arterioles and venules is observed at this stage with disappearance of the capillary net. The perivascular inflitrate of monocytes can still be present in the abnormal vessels at this time (Figure 1).

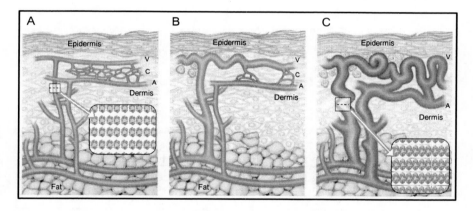

Figure 1. Evolution of a Cutaneous Telangiectasia in Hereditary Hemorrhagic Telangiectasia.**A**. In normal skin, arterioles (A) are connected to venules (V) through multiple capillaries (C). The ultrastructure of a normal postcapillary venule includes the lumen (L), endothelial cells, and two to three layers of surrounding pericytes. **B**. In the earliest stage of cutaneous telangiectasia, a single venule becomes dilated, but it is still connected to an arteriole through one or more capillaries. A perivascular lymphocytic infiltrate is apparent (asterisk). **C**. In a fully developed cutaneous telangiectasia, the venule has become markedly dilated throughout the dermis. The connecting arterioles have also become dilated and communicate directly with the venules without capillaries.The thickened wall of the dilated venules contains more than 10 layers of smooth-muscle cells. (Adapted from Gutmacher et al;1995).

HHT Is a Rare Disease in Spite of Its Autosomal Dominance

According to the literature it can be considered a rare disease as its prevalence ranges from 1:5000-8000 worldwid e[8]. It is calculated a population of 62500 affected individuals in Europe, and near one million people all over the world. However and due to a founder effect, there are certain areas with a higher prevalence. The most detailed study about prevalence of the disease was presented in 1989 by Plauchu et al., as a result of a research on French population concluding with a medium prevalence in France of 1/8,000 with higher rates in the Jurá area (1/2,351) [9]. The Dutch Antilles is the place with highest prevalence in the world (1/1,1331 in Curaçao and1/1,331 in Bonaire)[10]. Other areas with high concentration of cases are Akita in northern Japan (1/5,000-8,000) [11], the Fynn county in Denmark (1/1,641-7,246) [12], and more recently in Canary Islands (near 1/3,000) reported in the 10th HHT meeting in Cork (2013) (Table 1).

Table 1. Estimations of prevalence of HHT

Geographic Area	Prevalence	Reference
World estimation	1/5,000-8,000	Govani F et al. Eur J Hum Genet 2009; 17(7):860-871.
World estimation	min 1/10,000	Abdalla J et al. J Medical Genetics 2006; 43(2):97-110.
Europe estimation	1/5,000 - 8,000	Schoen FJ et al. Hum Mutat 2002; 19(2):140-148.
France	1/ 8,345	Plauchu et al. Am J. Med. Genet 1989; 32: 291-297.
Denmark	1/39,216	Kjeldsen AD et al. Chest 1999; 116(2):432-439.
Northern England	1/5,000 -8,000	Begbie ME et al. Postgrad Med J 2003; 79:18–24
Cantabria (Spain)	min 1:12,200	Morales C et al. Acta Otorrinolaring Esp. 1997; 48:625-629
Norway	1/8,000	Dheyauldeen S et al. Am J Rhinol Allergy 2011; 25(4):214-8
Netherlands	1:5,000-10,000.	Letteboer TG et al. Oral Pathol Oral Radiol Endod 2008; 105:38-41
Germany	1:10,000	Geisthoff UW et al. Arch Clin Exp Ophthalmol 2007; 245:1141-1144.
Italy	1/3,500-5,000	Sabbà et al. Minerva Cardiologica 2002; 50:221-238
USA	1/10,000	Guttmacher AE et al. N Engl J Med 2004; 351(22):2333-36
Vermont (USA)	1/16,500	Guttmacher AE et al. N Engl J Med 1995; 333:918
Japan	1/5,000 8,000	Dakeishi M et al. Hum Mutat 2002; 19(2):140-148.
Dutch Antilles	1/1,331	Jessurun GA et al. Clin Neurol Neurosurg 1993; 95(3):193-8
Funen (Denmark)	1/3,500	Kjeldsen AD et al. Chest 1999; 116(2):432-9

Table 2. Curaçao clinical criteria

1. Epistaxis	(Spontaneous and recurrent)
2. Telangiectases	(Multiple and in specific locations)
3. Dominant Inheritance Pattern	(a first-degree relative with HHT according to these criteria)
4. Internal Organ Involvement	(pulmonary, hepatic, cerebral, or spinal arteriovenous malformations, gastrointestinal telangiectasias)

HHT Clinical Diagnostic Criteria

Nose bleeding [13] is the main and earliest clinical symptom (90% of patients before the age of 21) present in more than 96% of patients. The epistaxis is also the circumstance affecting primarily the quality of life of HHT patients. However, there are certain cases where the pulmonary or the brain AVMs appear before the nose bleeding manifestation, in early ages, mainly children. Diagnosis is based on the clinical Curaçao criteria [14] (Table 2): epistaxis, mucocutaneous telangiectases in typical areas, family dominant pattern and internal organs involvement. Definite illness is diagnosed if three criteria are fulfilled and probable HHT if patient shows two of them. The identification of the causative mutation through molecular study is complementary to the probable or doubtful cases, and definite in relatives of affected families where the mutation for the index case is known. Penetrance is variable but in general it increases with age (90% at the age of 45) [15]. Due to the HHT rare condition, it is highly underdiagnosed all over the world, with a medium delay in diagnosis of patients estimated in about 30 years [16].

Clinical Symptoms

Although the most prevalent symptom is the epistaxis due to the rupture of local telangiectases in the nose, almost any organ of the body can be affected, occasionally with important associated morbi-mortality. In a study carried out on a Danish population of HHT patients [12] the mortality observed on HHT patients under 60 years old was higher than the expected for control population within the same age range. Pattern presentations are highly variable among families, even considering individuals of the same family. However, regarding genotype-phenotype correlation, pulmonary and brain AVMs have been observed with higher incidence on HHT type 1 patients, while HHT2 patients are in higher risk of gastrointestinal and hepatic involvement [17].

Epistaxis

The inspired air stream shear stress on the nasal mucose causes the rupture of these malformations with bleeding, present in more than 96% of patients. They normally constitute the earliest and more frequent manifestation of the disease. About 50% of HHT patients will present epistaxis before the age of 20. The Kiesselbach area is normally the most affected and usually the intensity increases with age. However sex, climate, diet, stress and pharmacological treatments can influence the frequency and quantity of nose bleeds [18].

There are several scales trying to quantify epistaxis severity: the Sadick scale [19] that considers frequency and quantity, and more recently the HHT epistaxis severity score (HHT-ESS) [20] that estimates frequency, quantity, characteristics of the bleeding, need for medical attention and the presence of anemia.

Mucocutaneous Telangiectases

They are present in more than 75% of HHT patients and appear normally from the second decade of life. They are usually round, 1-3 mms reddish spots that disappear with vitropression and normally located on lips, tongue, palate, fingers, face and ears (Figure 2).

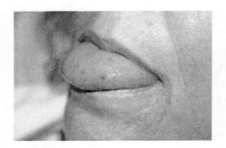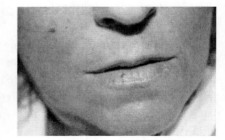

Figure 2. Typical telangiectases in HHT.

Apart from the presence of a mutation in heterozygous condition, it has been postulated the need for a "second hit" as physical trauma, wounds, or exposition to physical agents to trigger the telangiectases appearance. Due to the extinction of the capillary net and the arteriolization of the circulation, jet-bleedings are frequent when telangiectases break. Sometimes variations on the microscopic capillaries have been observed with a capillaroscopy [21] preceding the onset of macroscopic lesions, this circumstance which can be useful to clinically diagnose HHT in pediatric ages.

Pulmonary AVMs

It is estimated that 25-30% of HHT patients hold pulmonary arteriovenous malformations (PAVMs) while 90% of general patients with PAVMs suffer in fact from HHT. These arteriovenous malformations in the HHT lung patients are morphological and histologically indistinguishable from those present in non HHT ones; however PAVMs in HHT patients are more frequently multiple (35-65% of cases) and bilateral (25%) [22]. Pulmonary AVMs can be of two types: simple (80% of total, they have a unique afferent artery draining to a unique efferent vein through a bulbous, aneurismatic sac) and complex (20% of total, they have two or more subsegmentary afferent arteries connecting through an aneurismatic sac with two or more efferent arteries) [23]. Lesions are more frequent in lower pulmonary lobes due to dynamic blood flow and it is calculated that 25% of PAVMs grow gradually between 0.3 and 2 mm per year. This risk of enlargement is higher in adolescence, pregnancy and situations of high hypervolemia [24]. They can cause hypoxemia, rupture with secondary haemothorax or hemoptisis, paradoxical stroke (10-15% risk if not treated) due to right-left extracardiac shunting and central nervous system infections in case of paradoxical septic emboli [25]. Screening for PAVMs is mandatory in suspected or diagnosed HHT patients to prevent neurological complications that normally increase with age and number of lesions [25]. The most sensitive test to disclose PAVMs is cardiac echocardiography with agitated saline solution that can be graded to evaluate the possibility of finding large AVMs susceptible to be treated [26].

Hepatic AVMs

Although up to 75% of HHT patients will present liver involvement in image tests [27], it is normally asymptomatic (only 8% have severe symptoms associated with hepatic liver malformations (HAVMs), and characterized by the presence of telangiectases or confluent vascular structures, perfusion disturbances, enlargement of hepatic artery and venous-venous or portal-venous shunting. In cases of severe liver involvement and due to the double irrigation of the organ, we could find three types of shunts: arterio-hepatic (between hepatic artery and suprahepatic veins: these can lead to heart high-output failure), arterio-portal (between hepatic artery and porta vein: these can lead to cirrhosis) and porto-venous (between porta vein and suprahepatic veins) [28]. Heart failure is the most frequent manifestation of HAVMs (63%), portal hypertension occurs in 17% of severe cases and biliary ischemia in 19% of patients (normally associated with higher shunt grades). Other symptoms are portal-systemic encephalopathy (4%) and mesenteric ischemia. Liver biopsy is contraindicated in these patients (it must be considered also the highest prevalence of nodular focal hyperplasia due to HAVMs which can be confused with cirrotic nodules) and endoscopic cholangiography should be also avoided [29].

Brain AVMs

Between 10-20% of HHT patients present brain AVMs, representing a much higher incidence than the non HHT population. Lesions can range from telangiectases (40-50%), arteriovenous malformations (20%), to arteriovenous fistulae (20%), which represent direct connections between artery and vein with high flow, dural arteriovenous fistulae (5%) and cavernomatous malformations (5%)[30]. In HHT patients most lesions tend to be multiple (50% of individuals show two or more malformations)[31], with cortical location in almost all cases. Up to 23% of HHT patients present neurological symptoms as migraine, epilepsia, stroke, abscesses or hemorrhage[32]. Risk of bleeding remains controversial, with series that show less possibility compared with the general population (0.5% per year)[33], and others demonstrating over 20 times higher risks, depending on the type of vascular malformation[34] (normally lesions with deep venous drainage, unique drainage vein or high pressures on afferent arteries). Several cases of bleeding in newborn and young children have been described generally secondary to rupture of high flow pial fistulae. Screening with angio nuclear magnetic resonance is advisable at the moment of diagnosis of HHT and in newborns of parents with HHT and positive genetic test.

Spinal AVMs

Spinal cord lesions in HHT patients are perimedular intradural vascular malformations with direct connection between artery and vein and high flow[35]. They can be classified into micro and macro fistulae (the latter more frequent in HHT patients)[36]. The presence of a spinal macrofistula in paediatric ages could indicate suspected HHT. Symptomatology can be secondary to bleeding, compression, vascular robbery or venous thrombosis. Screening for spinal AVMs in young women could be indicated before pregnancy, or prior to delivery to prevent the punction of lesions in case of epidural anesthesia.

Gastrointestinal Bleeding

Gastrointestinal symptoms are related with the development of telangiectases in the digestive tract. These normally tend to appear from the fith-sixth decade of life and the presence of ferropenic anemia due to chronic bleeding is the rule. Although up to 80% of HHT patients can have lesions, only 13-33% present gastrointestinal bleeding[37] and symptoms can very often mistaken with swallowed blood from epistaxis. Digestive tract involvement is higher in the upper areas (stomach and first parts of the small bowell with normally multiple telangiectases) while the quantity of lesions present in jejunum and ileum correlate with the number of telangiectases present in duodenum[38]. Gastrointestinal tract involvement should be suspected when anemia is present in the—context of mild epistaxis and existence of telangiectases shown by endoscopic studies (gastroscopy, colonoscopy or videocapsule). Management is difficult mainly in distant telangiectases. Electrocoagulation of lesions should be only tried in a limited number of cases. Pharmacological management is similar to that used for nose bleeding. Surgery should be delayed as the last therapeutic solution for refractory bleeding. HHT patients with mutations in Smad 4 should be considered for early and periodical endoscopic screening to prevent development of local malignancy[39].

HHT Genetics

Considering molecular basis, two loci are involved by mutation in more than 90% of HHT cases. The first gene identified was *endoglin*, that maps to chromosome 9[40-42] and is responsible of 39-59% of the total HHT cases. Afterwards *ACVRL1* (activin like kinase type 1 or ALK1) was described[43,44], and maps to chromosome 12, being involved in 25%-57% of the HHT reports. Mutations in *ENG* and *ACVRL1* give rise to HHT1 and HHT2 types, respectively. In 2% of HHT patients the mutation is located in the *MADH4* gene (Smad4) leading to a combined syndrome of Juvenile familiar polyposis (JPHT) and HHT[45]. A third and fourth locus with a role in the genesis of HHT have been localized on chromosomes 5 and 7 with no identified genes, at the moment[46,47]. The pathogenical mechanism proposed for the HHT is the haploinsuficiency of endoglin, ALK1 or Smad 4[48,49]. The mutated counterpart gives rise to either RNA which suffers decay for a premature stop codon, codes for a protein which does not reach the membrane surface, or, even reaching the membrane, the product is functionally inactive in the TGF-β signaling cascade. In summary, the endothelial cell harbors only at the most, half of the functional protein (ENG, ALK1 or Smad4) and this amount is not enough to meet the physiological needs of the cell.

A geographical variation has been observed with higher prevalence of mutations in *ALK1* in the mediterranean regions[50,51] and on *Endoglin* in North America and Northern countries of Europe[52].

The mutations in *Endoglin* and *ALK1* are numerous, of different types including insertions, deletions, duplications, nucleotide changes, splice defects, loss of exons, and loss of the whole gene. The mutation database of Arup laboratories is in constant modification and with increasing number of mutations http://arup.utah.edu/database.

The three identified genes mutated in HHT (ACVRL1, ENG and MADH4) encode for proteins involved in the TGF-β signalling pathway[8].

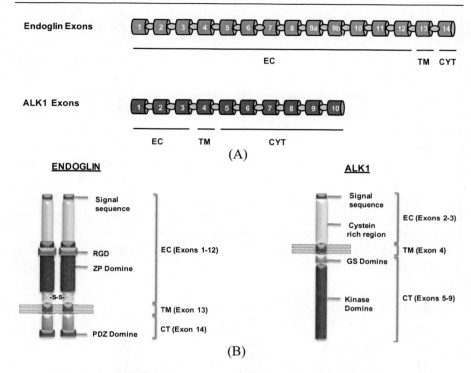

Figure 3. A. Schematic distribution of exons in *Endoglin* and *ACVRL1* genes (EC: extracellular domain, CYT: cytoplasmic domain, TM: transmembrane domain). **B.** Schematic distribution of different regions in Endoglin and ALK1 proteins.

Structure of Endoglin and ALK1

Both endoglin and ALK1 are type I trans-membrane proteins. The *Endoglin* gene is 40 kb long and was localized on chromosome 9q33-34 by linkage studies and *in situ* hybridization[40,41]. It is composed of 14 exons (exons 1 to 12 encode the extracellular domain, exon 13 encodes the transmembrane domain, and exon 14 encodes the cytoplasmic domain). On the other hand *ACVRL1* gene spans 13 Kb and mapped on 12q11-q14 and it is composed of 9 exons (exons 1 to 3 encode the extracellular domain, exon 4 encodes the transmembrane domain, and exon 5 to 10 encodes the cytoplasmic domain[43,44] (Figure 3A, 3B).

Endoglin is expressed as a 180-kDa disulfide-linked homodimer[53]. It contains a large extracellular domain of 561 amino acids, highly glycosylated mainly in asparagines residues. Structurally, endoglin belongs to the Zona

Pellucida (ZP) family of proteins that share a ZP domain of 260 amino acid residues at their extracellular region[54,55]. The third region does not show any significant homology to other protein family/domain and thereby has been named "orphan" domain. A transmembrane region, spanning 25 hydrophobic residues, acts as a linker between the ectodomain and the cytosolic region.

ALK1 is a transmembrane protein of approximately 55 kDa with an N-glycosylated ectodomain of 97 amino acids carrying a cysteine-rich small sequence which likely confers the appropriate structural conformation to capture the ligand. The ALK1 cytoplasmic region of 362 amino acids contains (i) a GS domain, a conserved 30 amino acids glycine/serine-rich sequence involved in the regulation of the receptor activation and (ii) a serine/threonine kinase domain. Phosphorylation of serine/threonine residues of ALK1 in the GS domain by the type II receptor (TβRII) leads to a conformational change in ALK1 that allows phosphorylation of the downstream signaling molecules Smad1, Smad5 or Smad8[56].

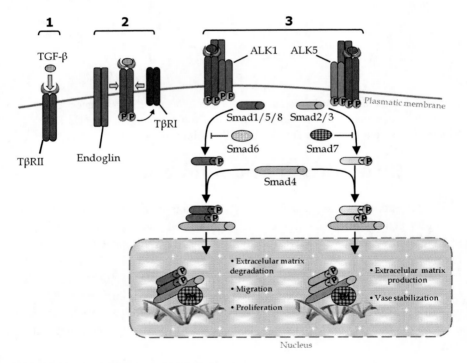

Figure 4. The TGF-β signaling pathway.

The TGF-β Pathway

Transforming growth factor-β1 (TGFβ-1) is the prototypic member of a large family of evolutionarily conserved pleiotropic secreted cytokines, which also includes the activins and bone morphogenetic proteins (BMPs). Individual family members have crucial roles in multiple processes throughout development and in the maintenance of tissue homeostasis in adult life[57]. Not surprisingly, therefore, subversion of signalling by TGFβ family members has been implicated in many human diseases, including cancer, fibrosis, autoimmune and vascular diseases[58-60].

TGF-β signals through a heteromeric complex of type I (RI) and type II (RII) which are transmembrane serine/threonine kinase receptors (Figure 4). Although the core of the TGF-β receptor complex is formed by the association of RI and RII, it may also contain auxiliary receptors such as endoglin and betaglycan.

First, TGF-β binds RII with a high affinity. This TGF-β/RII complex then recruits RI. Once the heteromeric complex TGF-β/RII/RI is formed, a domain of RI is phosphorylated by RII[57,61]. This phosphorylation of serine/threonine residues leads to RI activation, in turn propagating the signal through a cascade of intracellular effectors which belong to the Smad protein family. There are three different types of Smads: receptor regulated (R-Smads), common mediator (Co-Smads) and inhibitory (I-Smads) Smads. R-Smads like Smad1, Smad2, Smad3, Smad5 and Smad8 are phosphorylated and activated by RI and these activated R-Smads bind subsequently to the Co-Smad, Smad4. The R-Smad/Co-Smad complexes translocate to the nucleus where they contribute to the transcriptional activation of target genes[62]. The I-Smads (Smad6 and Smad7) prevent R-Smad phosphorylation by competing with R-Smads for receptor interaction through recruitment of ubiquitin ligases to the activated receptor leading to its proteosomal degradation, or by recruiting phosphatases that inactivate RI[63,64] (Figure 4).

Several members of the TGF-β superfamily, including TGF-β1, TGF-β3, activin-A, BMP-2, BMP-7 and BMP-9 are able to bind endoglin and/or ALK1. This binding triggers the Smad-dependent downstream signaling[65,66].

In ECs, endoglin modulates ligand binding and signaling by association with ALK1 and ALK5[65-68]. Thus, endoglin inhibits the TGF-β/ALK5/Smad3-mediated cellular responses such as the increased expression of the plasminogen activator inhibitor 1 (PAI-1). By contrast, endoglin promotes the ALK5/Smad2-mediated upregulation of endothelial nitric oxide synthase (eNOS) as well as the TGF-β1/ALK1-mediated increase of Id1.

Interestingly, endoglin inhibits the BMP-9/ALK1 signalling in ECs. Overall, endoglin appears to be a critical modulator of the balance between ALK1 and ALK5 signaling[69-71].

Different studies support the view that endoglin and ALK1 participate in a common signaling pathway that is critical for EC responses to TGF-β family members[70-72]. This conclusion agrees with the fact that pathogenic mutations in *ENG* or *ACVRL1* genes result in HHT and that ALK1 and endoglin null mice have similar vascular phenotypes[73].

Functional Implications of Endoglin and ALK1

Endoglin and ALK1 are expressed in endothelial cells (ECs), which are the primary cell target in HHT. Endoglin is expressed at low levels in resting ECs, but at high levels in endothelial proliferating cells at sites of active angiogenesis and during embryogenesis[72]. Other cell types that express endoglin at their surface are macrophages, erythroid precursors in bone marrow, syncytiotrophoblasts and several cell types closely related to the cardiovascular system such as smooth muscle cells of atherosclerotic plaques and cardiac fibroblasts[71].

Upregulated expression of endoglin was found in inflamed or infected tissues, healing wounds, psoriatic skin, synovial arthritis, upon vascular injury and in tumoral vessels[71,74,75]. Under hypoxic conditions, the hypoxia inducible factor-1 (HIF-1) complex binds a functional consensus hypoxia responsive element (HRE) in the ENG gene promoter[76]. TGF-β signaling, via Smad transcription factors, also potently stimulates endoglin expression[77,78]. Whereas hypoxia alone moderately stimulates endoglin transcription, addition of TGF-β1 under hypoxic conditions results in a transcriptional cooperation between both signalling pathways, leading to a marked stimulation of endoglin expression. This synergic stimulation involves the formation of a transcriptional multicomplex containing Smad3/Smad4, Sp1, and HIF-1[76]. Upon vascular injury, a transcriptional activation of endoglin mediated by the cooperative interaction between Sp1 and KLF6 transcription factors has been reported[74].By contrast, tumor necrosis factor-alpha (TNF-α) decreases endoglin protein levels in ECs[71].

Endoglin is also implicated in the cytoskeletal organization. The cytoplasmic tail of L-endoglin interacts with members of the LIM domain-containing family of proteins, including zyxin and ZRP-1 (zyxin-related protein-1), involved in regulating cytoskeleton, assembly and cell motility[79]. The organization of the capillary network during angiogenesis depends on the structure of ECs so that in the vasculature of HHT patients a disorganized cytoskeleton is prone to cell breaking with changes in shear stress and blood pressure. This might lead to vessel haemorrhages and eventual disappearance of the capillary network, as occurs in HHT[80].

On the other hand, expression of endoglin in the tumor cells appears to play an important role in the progression of cancer, influencing cell proliferation, motility, invasiveness and tumorigenicity[72,81,82]. In addition, in vitro and in vivo experiments in which endoglin expression is modulated, have provided evidence supporting endoglin as a tumor suppressor[83]. Interestingly, increased levels of soluble endoglin have been detected in plasma, serum and urine from patients with different pathologies, including preeclampsia and cancer[72]. This soluble endoglin comes from a proteolytic shedding of the membrane bound protein. MT-1 is the metaloprotease responsible for the cleavage[84]. Circulating soluble endoglin is a reliable marker of preeclampsia and is associated with poor prognosis in cancer. Whereas it has been postulated a pathogenic role for soluble endoglin in preeclampsia due to its anti-angiogenic activity, the role of soluble endoglin in tumor progression remains to be established[83]. Decreased levels of soluble endoglin have been detected in plasma samples of HHT patients, as a reflect of decreased endoglin on the membrane surface[85].

ALK1 expression has been reported not only in highly vascularized tissues including lung, placenta, and heart, but also at specific sites of epithelial-mesenchymal interactions, and in other cell types such as monocytes, microglia, skin fibroblasts, stellate hepatic cells, chondrocytes, neural crest stem cells and more recently myoblasts[67,71]. Nonetheless, most studies to date suggest that its major roles are related to the endothelial specific expression pattern. ALK1 is involved in angiogenesis and a regulatory region of ACVRL1 gene is sufficient for endothelial expression in arteries feeding ischemic tissues[86]. The characterization of ACVRL1 promoter and the study of its transcriptional regulation has begun to be elucidated by Garrido-Martín et al. (2011) and its transcriptional activation upon vascular injury, through Sp1 and KLF6 cooperation has been recently described[87].

General Clinical Recommendations for Management of HHT Patients

Given the risk of multisystemic affectation in HHT patients, the international guidelines[88] recommend the performance of a screening protocol to disclose the presence of internal organ involvement. These protocols are in constant revision due to the appearance of new evidences but they constitute a very appropriate initial approach to the correct management of the disease. Although, there is a lack of wide series and clinical trials, due to the rare character of the disease, and differences regarding health systems, experts recommend to perform in adults a routine blood test, genetic test if available (to identify the causative mutation, cardiac echocardiography with contrast (if positive, a computed tomography scan to identify pulmonary AVMs and subsequent diagnostic/therapeutic angiography), liver doppler ultrasound study, brain angio-magnetic resonance and ENT evaluation. In case of children, this screening protocol tries to disclose brain AVMs (angio-magnetic resonance) and if the child is asymptomatic, pulmonary screening could be delayed till adolescence.

Treatment

There is not a definite treatment for HHT and due to its quality of rare disease and the lack of normalized clinical trials, the support therapies either pharmacological, surgical or combination of both are based in the "state of the art" practice.

Epistaxis

The pharmacological handling of the nose bleeding, almost similar as in the case of gastrointestinal bleeding, and in addition to the general measures of local moisturing, tamponage (preferably with neumatic or autodissolving devices) and iron supplies in case of anemia, relies on six possible alternatives:

1. **Antifibrinolytic therapy**: ε-aminocaproic and mainly tranexamic acid[89], locally inhibitors of the fibrinolysis on the wall of the telangiectases with stabilization of the clot and, as *in vitro* observed,

increase of the quantity of endoglin and transcriptional induction of endoglin and ALK1 mRNA[80]. A clinical trial has been carried out showing decrease in frequency and quantity of nose bleeding with 1.5 g/day of oral tranexamic acid[90].

2. **Antiangiogenic therapy**: the vascular endothelial growth factors (VEGFs) are specific mitogens for vascular endothelial cells and essential in the process of angiogenesis and lymphangiogenesis in most of physiological and pathological conditions. Some series of cases have been reported about improvement of nose bleeding in HHT with bevacizumab, a recombinant humanized monoclonal antibody to VEGF-A ligand, both topical and systemic, but with no long-term effect is observed after its removal[91-93]. Also thalidomide, a suppressor of several cytokines and angiogenic factors (VEGF, TNF-α and interleukine 6) has been shown to improve nose bleeding in short series of HHT patients[94] and also in non HHT patients with angiodysplasias in the gastrointestinal tract[95].

3. **Immunosupressant drugs**: several cases of HHT patients treated with sirolimus or tacrolimus due to concomitant pathology (transplants) showed improvement on bleeding severity[96]. This effect is likely due to a promoter increase of *ENG* and *ALK1* TGF-β pathway dependent[97].

4. **Anti-oxidant agents**, such as N-acetylcysteine. In a pilot study developed on 43 HHT patients treated daily with 600 mg/day of N-acetylcisteine for an average of 11 weeks, nose bleeding decreased[98,99].

5. **Hormonal treatment**: hormonal therapy with ethynilestradiol alone or combined with progesterone can be useful to alleviate nose and gastrointestinal bleeding in HHT patients[100]. Also danazol seems to have similar results and to be better for male HHT population to avoid estrogenic feminizing side effects[101]. Based on results with tamoxifen on HHT women with breast cancer and on series of patients that showed improvement in bleeding severity[102,103], a study with raloxifene (a selective estrogen receptor modulator indicated for treatment and prevention of postmenopausal osteoporosis and with advantages on cardiovascular profile and prevention of breast cancer), was carried out on postmenopausal HHT women with HHT at a dose of 60 mgrs./day. After a medium period of 18 months 72% of patients improved symptoms considering frequency and quantity of epistaxis. In parallel, molecular bases of raloxifene effects on cells were studied,

concluding that raloxifene binds the promotor of endoglin and ALK1, estimulating their transcription[104]. With these data, raloxifene was designed as the first orphan drug for HHT by the European Medicines Agency and the Food and Drug Administration in 2009 (EMEA/OD/ 138/09, EU/3/10/730, FDA/10/3099).

6. Other approaches have been performed with propranolol, a β-blocker that is currently considered the most efficient drug treatment for the infantile haemangiomas. Antiangiogenic properties of propranolol have been tested in endothelial cells to check the availability for topical use in HHT patients showing its capacity to decrease cellular migration and tube formation and also apoptotic effects[105]. Isolate reports with other drugs such as bleomycin have been presented with variable results.

It must be considered the fact that most of the previously cited treatment options (mainly hormonal treatment, antifibrynolytics and antiangiogenics) could lead as a side effect to thromboembolism phenomena. There are reports on HHT patients that show high amounts of VIII coagulation factor and an increased number of deep venous thrombosis and pulmonary thromboembolism[106], so careful estimation of risk-benefit must be considered when taking in consideration the use of any of them. On the other hand in HHT patients with atrial fibrillation or prostetic heart valves or any circumstance with the necessity or option to be treated with antiplatelets or anticoagulants, risk-benefit should be considered prior being this circumstance a relative but not absolute contraindication for its administration.

In case of failing of the pharmacological approach or impossibility of its administration, a surgical approach (combined with systemic drugs or alone) should be considered. The possibilities in this field can be "minor surgery": electrocoagulation of the local lesions with argon plasma[107] or laser combined or not with topical estrogens or local injection of bevacizumab[108]; local sclerotherapy with ethoxysclerol that has been proved to be a good option in patients with mild-moderate bleeding[109] or "major surgery": septodermoplasty[110] with a substitution of the damaged mucosa by a cutaneous implant (it normally improves the clinic but many patients refer dryness and bad smell); nostrils closure[111] has been shown in some series to be a good option and quite well tolerated. Supraselective embolization of maxilary artery branches is reserved only for cases of unstoppable bleeding or preparation for additional techniques as its effects is normally very short in time.

Pulmonary AVMs

In the case of adult patients with HHT and pulmonary arteriovenous malformations, embolization[112] of lesions, even if they are diffuse[113], is recommended (with coils or Amplatzer devices) to reduce the potential risk of paradoxical stroke and septic paradoxical embolism. Malformations with an afferent artery over 3mm where supposed to be in a higher risk of complications but recent articles postulate that risk does not depend on this size and all accessible lesions should be treated[114]. Follow up after treatment is based on computer tomography studies and recommended in the next 6-12 months. In the paediatric population, management is different as the risk of stroke is lower and in most cases if the patient is asymptomatic, treatment is delayed until puberty[115]. All patients with pulmonary AVMs, treated or not, should receive antibiotic profilaxis in case of procedures with risk of bacteremia, mainly of the bucal area, to prevent development of abscesses[116]. Pulmonary hypertension has been related in some cases with ALK1 mutations but in most cases of HHT it is secondary to liver/heart failure, and it must be managed currently[117].

Liver AVMs

Although more than 70% of HHT patients can present liver involvement, only 8% show symptoms. Pharmacological management of clinical symptomatology associated with high-output heart failure, cirrhosis and cholangitis is the initial measure but in severe cases liver transplantation has been proved the alternative with the highest survival rates[118]. Other alternatives as hepatic artery embolization appear to have higher morbi-mortality rates and worse survival prediction. Some trials with antiangiogenics (bevacizumab) mainly in cases of heart failure have been performed with good outcomes[119]. Follow-up of liver affected HHT patients show the need to undergo a close control mainly for cases with hepatic AVMs as there is favourable response to treatment (either pharmacological/surgical) in 63% of cases and indicating the heart failure and the development of arrythmias as the most associated symptoms[120].

Brain AVMs

Cerebral arteriovenous malformations when disclosed can be managed as in non HHT patients with embolisation, stereotactic radiation and surgery or combinations of previous[121,122]. There are not long-term results on wide series of these patients and recommendations relay on the need of expertise for the management of these patients and to treat in prevention those lesions with higher risk to bleed (i.e. high-flow pial fistulae). Cerebral abscesses in HHT patients are mostly related with the presence of pulmonary AVMs and normally caused by anaerobious bacteria (mainly Streptococcus); they must be treated as in non HHT patients (antibiotics and/or surgery)[123].

Pregnancy

Most of deliveries in HHT pregnant women proceed normally, however, due to dynamic blood flow specific circumstances pregnancy is in a higher risk of enlargement of pulmonary AVMs and bleeding[124], cardiac heart failure[125], epistaxis and mucose telangiectases worsening due to the hormonal natural state while there is no evidence about management of brain AVMs during pregnancy, recommending the guidelines to wait till delivery to perform the specific treatment if needed in this case. Recognition of the HHT condition and the presence of pulmonary AVMs before pregnancy increases rates of survival however pregnant HHT women should be treated as high risk obstetric patients[126].

Pediatrics and HHT

There is no evidence about HHT increased risk for birth defects[127], however a high prevalence of arteriovenous malformations have been disclosed in children at early ages or even at birth[128] bringing on the table the necessity of check up at this age. Screening for asymptomatic HHT children is under debate but due to the potentially life-threatening manifestations should be considered mainly for brain AVMs[129].

References

[1]   Sutton, H. Epistaxis as an indication of impaired nutrition, and of degeneration of the vascular system. *Med Mirror*, 1864, 769-81.

[2]   Rendu, H. Épistaxis répeteés chez un sujet porteur de petits angiomes cutanees et muqueux. *Gaz Hop*, 1896, 1322-3.

[3]   Osler, W. On a family form of recurring epistaxis, associated with multiple telangiectases of the skin and mucous membranes. *Bull Johns Hopkins Hops*, 1901, 12, 333-7.

[4]   Weber, F. Multiple hereditary developmental angiomata (telangiectases) of the skin and mucous membranes associated with recurring haemorrhages. *Lancet*, 1907, 2, 160-2.

[5]   Hanes, F. Multiple hereditary telangiectases causing hemorrhage (hereditary hemorrhagic telangiectasia). *Bull Johns Hopkins Hosp*, 1909, 20, 63-73.

[6]   Ikawa, T; Tokunaga, T; Matsumura, M; Imayama, S. An electron microscopic study in Osler´s disease. *J Clin Electron Microscopy*, 1983, 16, 5-6

[7]   Jahnke, V. Ultraestructure of hereditary telangiectasia. *Arch Otolaryng*, 1970, 91, 262-5.

[8]   Govani, FS; Shovlin, CL. Hereditary hemorrhagic telangiectasia:a clinical and scientific review. *Eur J Hum Genet*, 2009, 17(7), 860-71.

[9]   Plauchu, H; de Chadarévian, JP; Bideau, A; Robert, JM. Age-related clinical profile of hereditary hemorrhagic telangiectasia in an epidemiologically recruited population. *Am J Med Genet*, 1989, 32, 291-7.

[10]   Jessurum, GA; Kamphuis, DJ; van der, Zande, FH; Nossent, JC. Cerebral arteriovenous malformations in the Netherlands Antilles;high prevalence of hereditary hemorrhagic telangiectasia-related single and multiple cerebral arteriovenous malformations. *Clin Neurol Neurosurg*, 1993, 95(3), 193-8.

[11]   Dakeishi, M; Shioya, T; Wada, Y; et al. Genetic epidemiology of hereditary hemorrhagic telangiectasia in a local community in the northern part of Japan. *Hum Mutat*, 2002, 19(2), 140-148.

[12]   Kjeldsen, AD; Vase, P; Green, A. Hereditary hemorrhagic telangiectasia:a population-based study of prevalence and mortality in Danish patients. *J Intern Med*, 1999, 245(1), 31-9.

[13]   Os, AA; Friedman, CM; White, RI, Jr. The natural history of epistaxis in hereditary hemorrhagic telangiectasia. *Laryngoscope*, 1991, 101, 977-80

[14] Shovlin, CL; Guttmacher, AE; Buscarini, E; et al. Diagnostic criteria for hereditary hemorrhagic telangiectasia (Rendu Osler Weber syndrome). *Am J Genet*, 2000, 91, 66-7.

[15] Guttmacher, AE; Marchuuk, DA; White, RI, Jr. Hereditary hemorrhagic telangiectasia. *N Engl J Med*, 1995, 333, 918-24.

[16] Pierucci, P; Lenato, GM; Suppressa, P; et al. A long diagnostic delay in patients with hereditary hemorrhagic telangiectasia:a questionnaire-based retrospective study. *Orphanet J rare Dis*, 2012, 7, 33.

[17] Lesca, G; Olivieri, C; Burnichon, N; et al. Genotype-phenotype correlations in hereditary hemorrhagic telangiectasia, data from the French-Italian HHT network. *Genet Med*, 2007, 9, 14-22.

[18] Aassar, O; Friedman, C; White, R. The natural history of epistaxis in hereditary hemorrhagic telangiectasia. *Laryngoscope*, 1991, 101, 977-80.

[19] Sadick, H; Naim, R; Oulmi, J; et al. Plasma surgery and topical estriol, effects on the nasal mucosa and long-term results in patients with Osler´s disease. *Otolaryngol Head Neck Surg*, 2003, 129, 233-8.

[20] Hoag, JB; Terry, P; Mitchell, S; et al. An epistaxis severity score for hereditary hemorrhagic telangiectasia. *Laryngoscope* 2010, 120, 838-43.

[21] Mager, JJ; Westermann, CJ. Value of capillary microscopy in the diagnosis of hereditary hemorrhagic telangiectasia. *Arch Dermatol*, 2000, 136, 732-4.

[22] White, RI; Mitchell, SE; Barth, KH; et al. Angioarchitecture of pulmonary arteriovenous malformations:an important consideration before embolotherapy. *Am J Roentgenol*, 1983, 140, 681-6.

[23] Gossage, JR; Kanj, G. Pulmonary arteriovenous malformations. A state of the art review. *Am J Respir Crit Care Med*, 1998, 158, 643-61.

[24] Dines, D; Arms, R; Bernatz, P; et al. Pulmonary arteriovenous fistulas. *Mayo Clin Proc*, 1974, 49, 460-5.

[25] McDonald, J; Bayrak-Toydemir, P; Pyeritz, RE. Hereditary hemorrhagic telangiectasia:an overview of diagnosis, management and pathogenesis. *Genet Med*, 2011, 7, 607-16.

[26] Parra, JA; Bueno, J; Zarauza, J; et al. Graded contrast echocardiography in pulmonary arteriovenous malformations. *Eur Respir J*, 2010, 35, 1-7.

[27] Ianora, AAS; memeo, M; Sabba, C et al. Multi-detector Row Helical CT assessment of hepatic involvement. *Radiology*, 2004, 230, 250-9.

[28] García-Tsao, G; Korzenik, JR; Young, L; et al. Liver disease in patients with hereditary hemorrhagic telangiectasia. *N Engl J Med*, 2000, 343, 931-6.

[29] Buscarini, E; Danesino, C; Plauchu, H; et al. High prevalence of hepatic focal nodular hyperplasia in subjects with hereditary hemorrhagic telangiectasia. *Ultrasound in Medicine & biology*, 2004, 30, 1089-97.

[30] Matsubara, S; Manzia, JL; Ter, Brugge, K; et al. Angiographic and clinical characteristics of patients with cerebral arteriovenous malformations associated with hereditary hemorrhagic telangiectasia. *AJNR Am J Neuroradiol*, 2000, 21, 1016-20.

[31] Dowd, CF; William, L; Ter Brugge, K; et al. Quantitative assesment brain arteriovenous malformation multiplicity predicts the diagnosis of hereditary hemorrhagic telangiectasia. *Stroke*, 2012, 43, 72-78.

[32] Nishida, T; Faughnam, ME; Krings, T; et al. Brain arteriovenous malformations associated with hereditary hemorrhagic telangiectasia: gene-phenotype correlations. *Am J Med Genet A*, 2012, 158, 2829-34.

[33] McDonald, R; Stoodley, M; Weir, B. Vascular malformations of the central nervous system. *Neurosurgery Quaterly*, 2001, 11, 231-47.

[34] Easey, AJ; Wallace, GMF; Hugues, JMB; et al. Should asymptomatic patients with hereditary hemorrhagic telangiectasia (HHT) be screened for cerebral vascular malformations? Data from 22061 years of patient life. *J Neurol Neurosurg Psychiatry*, 2003, 74, 743-8.

[35] Cullen, S; Alvarez, H; Rodesch, G; et al. Spinal arteriovenous shunts presenting before 2 years of age, analysis of 13 cases. *Child's Nervous System*, 2006, 22, 1103-10.

[36] Rodesch, G; Hurth, M; Alvarez, H; et al. Classification of spinal cord arteriovenous shunts, proposal for a reappraisal:the Bicetre experience with 155 consecutive patients treated between 1981 and 1999. *Neurosurg*, 2002, 51, 374-80.

[37] Kjeldsen, AD; Kjeldsen, J. Gastrointestinal bleeding in patients with hereditary hemorrhagic telangiectasia. *Am J Gastroenterol*, 2000, 95, 415-8.

[38] Proctor, DD; Henderson, KZ; Dziura, JD; et al. Enteroscopic evaluation of the gastrointestinal tract in symptomatic patients with hereditary hemorrhagic telangiectasia. *J Clin Gastroenterol*, 2005, 39, 115-9.

[39] Schwenter, F; Faughnam, ME; Gradinger, AB; et al. Juvenile polyposis, hereditary hemorrhagic telangiectasia and early onset colorectal cancer in patients with SMAD4 mutation. *J Gastroenterol*, 2012, 47, 795-804.

[40] McDonald, MT; Papenberg, KA; Ghosh, S; Glatfelter, AA; Biesecker, BB; Helmbold, EA; Markel, DS; Zolotor, A; McKinnon, WC; Vanderstoep, JL; Jackson, CE; Iannuzzi, M; Collins, FS; Boehnke, M; Porteous, ME; Guttmacher, AE, y; Marchuk, DA. A disease locus for

hereditary haemorrhagic telangiectasia maps to chromosome 9q33-34. *Nat Genet*, 1994, 6, 197-204.

[41] Fernandez-Ruiz, E; St-Jacques, S; Bellon, T; Letarte, M, y; Bernabeu, C. Assignment of the human endoglin gene (END) to 9q34-->qter. *Cytogenet Cell Genet*, 1993, 64, 204-7.

[42] McAllister, KA; Grogg, KM; Johnson, DW; Gallione, CJ; Baldwin, MA; Jackson, CE; Helmbold, EA; Markel, DS; McKinnon, WC; Murrell, J; McCormick, MK; Pericak-Vance, MA; Heutink, P; Oostra, BA; Haitjema, T; Westerman, CJJ; Porteous, ME; Guttmacher, AE; Letarte, M, y; Marchuk, DA. Endoglin, a TGF-beta binding protein of endothelial cells, is the gene for hereditary haemorrhagic telangiectasia type 1. *Nat Genet*, 1994, 8, 345-51.

[43] Johnson, DW; Berg, JN; Baldwin, MA; Gallione, CJ; Marondel, I; Yoon, SJ; Stenzel, TT; Speer, M; Pericak-Vance, MA; Diamond, A; Guttmacher, AE; Jackson, CE; Attisano, L; Kucherlapati, R; Porteous, ME, y; Marchuk, DA. Mutations in the activin receptor-like kinase 1 gene in hereditary haemorrhagic telangiectasia type 2. *Nat Genet*, 1996, 13, 189-95.

[44] Johnson, DW; Berg, JN; Gallione, CJ; McAllister, KA; Warner, JP; Helmbold, EA; Markel, DS; Jackson, CE; Porteous, ME y; Marchuk, DA. A second locus for hereditary hemorrhagic telangiectasia maps to chromosome 12. *Genome research*, 1995, 5, 21-8.

[45] Gallione, CJ; Repetto, GM; Legius, E; Rustgi, AK; Schelley, SL; Tejpar, S; Mitchell, G; Drouin, E; Westermann, CJ y; Marchuk, DA. A combined syndrome of juvenile polyposis and hereditary haemorrhagic telangiectasia associated with mutations in MADH4 (SMAD4). *Lancet*, 2004, 363, 852-9.

[46] Cole, SG; Begbie, ME; Wallace, GM, y; Shovlin, CL. A new locus for hereditary haemorrhagic telangiectasia (HHT3) maps to chromosome 5. *J Med Genet*, 2005, 42, 577-82.

[47] Bayrak-Toydemir, P; McDonald, J; Akarsu, N; Toydemir, RM; Calderon, F; Tuncali, T; Tang, W; Miller, F, y; Mao, R. A fourth locus for hereditary hemorrhagic telangiectasia maps to chromosome 7. *Am J Med Genet*, 2006, 140, 2155-62.

[48] Marchuk, DA. Genetic abnormalities in hereditary hemorrhagic telangiectasia. *Curr Opin Hematol*, 1998, 5, 332-8.

[49] Shovlin, CL. Molecular defects in rare bleeding disorders, hereditary haemorrhagic telangiectasia. *Thromb Haemost*, 1997, 78, 145-50.

[50] Fernandez-L, A; Sanz-Rodriguez, F; Zarrabeitia, R; Perez-Molino, A; Morales, C; Restrepo, CM; Ramirez, JR; Coto, E; Lenato, GM; Bernabeu, C, y; Botella, LM. Mutation study of Spanish patients with hereditary hemorrhagic telangiectasia and expression analysis of Endoglin and ALK1. *Hum Mutat*, 2006, 27, 295.

[51] Olivieri, C; Mira, E; Delu, G; Pagella, F; Zambelli, A; Malvezzi, L; Buscarini, E, y; Danesino, C. Identification of 13 new mutations in the ACVRL1 gene in a group of 52 unselected Italian patients affected by hereditary haemorrhagic telangiectasia. *J Med Genet*, 2002, 39, E39.

[52] Abdalla, SA; Pece-Barbara, N; Vera, S; Tapia, E; Paez, E; Bernabeu, C, y; Letarte, M. Analysis of ALK-1 and endoglin in newborns from families with hereditary hemorrhagic telangiectasia type 2. *Hum Mol Genet*, 2000, 9, 1227-37.

[53] Gougos, A, y; Letarte, M. Primary structure of endoglin, an RGD-containing glycoprotein of human endothelial cells. *J Biol Chem*, 1990, 265, 8361-4.

[54] Jovine, L; Darie, CC; Litscher, ES; Wassarman, PM. Zona pellucida domain proteins. *Annu Rev Biochem*, 2005, 74, 83-114.

[55] Llorca, O; Trujillo, A; Blanco, FJ; Bernabeu, C. Structural model of human endoglin, a transmembrane receptor responsible for hereditary hemorrhagic telangiectasia. *J Mol Biol*, 2007, 365,694-705.

[56] Gordon, KJ; Blobe, GC. Role of transforming growth factor-beta superfamily signaling pathways in human disease. *Biochim Biophys Acta*, 2008, 1782, 197-228.

[57] Massague, J. TGF-beta signal transduction. *Annu Rev Biochem*, 1998, 67, 753-91.

[58] Pardali, E; Goumans, MJ, y; ten, Dijke, P. Signaling by members of the TGF-beta family in vascular morphogenesis and disease. *Trends Cell Biol*, 2010, 20, 556-67.

[59] Van, Meeteren, LA, y; Ten, Dijke, P. Regulation of endothelial cell plasticity by TGF-beta. *Cell Tissue Res*, 2011, 347, 177-86.

[60] Bobik, A. Transforming growth factor-betas and vascular disorders. *Arterioscler Thromb Vasc Biol*, 2006, 26, 1712-20.

[61] Wieser, R; Wrana, JL, y; Massague, J. GS domain mutations that constitutively activate T beta R-I, the downstream signaling component in the TGF-beta receptor complex. *EMBO J*, 1995, 14, 2199-208.

[62] Massague, J; Seoane, J, y; Wotton, D. Smad transcription factors. *Genes Dev*, 2005, 19, 2783-810.

[63] Itoh, S, y; ten, Dijke, P. Negative regulation of TGF-beta receptor/Smad signal transduction. *Curr Opin Cell Biol*, 2007, 19, 176-84.

[64] Valdimarsdottir, G; Goumans, MJ; Itoh, F; Itoh, S; Heldin, CH, y; ten, Dijke, P. Smad7 and protein phosphatase 1alpha are critical determinants in the duration of TGF-beta/ALK1 signaling in endothelial cells. *BMC Cell Biol*, 2006, 7, 16.

[65] Guerrero-Esteo, M; Sanchez-Elsner, T; Letamendia, A, y; Bernabeu, C. Extracellular and cytoplasmic domains of endoglin interact with the transforming growth factor-beta receptors I and II. *J Biol Chem*, 2002, 277, 29197-209.

[66] Blanco, FJ; Santibañez, JF; Guerrero-Esteo, M; Langa, C; Vary, CP, y; Bernabeu, C. Interaction and functional interplay between endoglin and ALK-1, two components of the endothelial transforming growth factor-beta receptor complex. *J Cell Physiol*, 2005, 204, 574-84.

[67] Velasco, S; Alvarez-Muñoz, P; Pericacho, M; Dijke, PT; Bernabéu, C; López-Novoa, JM; Rodríguez-Barbero, A. L-and S-endoglin differentially modulate TGFbeta1 signaling mediated by ALK1 and ALK5 in L6E9 myoblasts. *J Cell Sci*, 2008, 121, 913-919.

[68] Santibañez, JF; Letamendia, A; Perez-Barriocanal, F; Silvestri, C; Saura, M; Vary, CP; Lopez-Novoa, JM; Attisano, L, y; Bernabeu, C. Endoglin increases eNOS expression by modulating Smad2 protein levels and Smad2-dependent TGF-beta signaling. *J Cell Physiol*, 2007, 210, 456-68.

[69] David, L; Feige, JJ; Bailly, S. Emerging role of bone morphogenetic proteins in angiogenesis. *Cytokine Growth Factor Rev*, 2009, 20, 203-212.

[70] Lebrin, F; Mummery, CL. Endoglin-mediated vascular remodeling: mechanisms underlying hereditary hemorrhagic telangiectasia. *Trends Cardiovasc Med*, 2008, 18, 25-32.

[71] Bernabeu, C; Conley, BA; Vary, CP. Novel biochemical pathways of endoglin in vascular cell physiology. *J Cell Biochem*, 2007, 102, 1375-1388.

[72] Bernabeu, C; Lopez-Novoa, JM, y; Quintanilla, M. The emerging role of TGF-beta superfamily coreceptors in cancer. *Biochim Biophys Acta*, 2009, 1792, 954-73.

[73] Abdalla, SA, y; Letarte, M. Hereditary haemorrhagic telangiectasia, current views on genetics and mechanisms of disease. *J Med Genet*, 2006, 43, 97-110.

[74] Botella, LM; Sanchez-Elsner, T; Sanz-Rodriguez, F; Kojima, S; Shimada, J; Guerrero-Esteo, M; Cooreman, MP; Ratziu, V; Langa, C; Vary, CP; Ramirez, JR; Friedman, S, y; Bernabeu, C. Transcriptional activation of endoglin and transforming growth factor-beta signaling components by cooperative interaction between Sp1 and KLF6, their potential role in the response to vascular injury. *Blood*, 2002, 100, 4001-10.

[75] Fonsatti, E; Nicolay, HJ; Altomonte, M; Covre, A; Maio, M. Targeting cancer vasculature via endoglin/cd105:a novel antibody-based diagnostic and therapeutic strategy in solid tumors. *Cardiovasc Res*, 2010, 86(1), 12-9.

[76] Sanchez-Elsner, T; Botella, LM; Velasco, B; Langa, C, y; Bernabeu, C. Endoglin expression is regulated by transcriptional cooperation between the hypoxia and transforming growth factor-beta pathways. *J Biol Chem*, 2002, 277, 43799-808.

[77] Botella, LM; Sanchez-Elsner, T; Rius, C; Corbi, A, y; Bernabeu, C. Identification of a critical Sp1 site within the endoglin promoter and its involvement in the transforming growth factor-beta stimulation. *J Biol Chem*, 2001, 276, 34486-94.

[78] Rius, C; Smith, JD; Almendro, N; Langa, C; Botella, LM; Marchuk, DA; Vary, CP, y; Bernabeu, C. Cloning of the promoter region of human endoglin, the target gene for hereditary hemorrhagic telangiectasia type 1. *Blood*, 1998, 92, 4677-90.

[79] Sanz-Rodriguez, F; Guerrero-Esteo, M; Botella, LM; Banville, D; Vary, CP, y; Bernabeu, C. Endoglin regulates cytoskeletal organization through binding to ZRP-1, a member of the Lim family of proteins. *J Biol Chem*, 2004, 279, 32858-68.

[80] Fernandez-L, A; Garrido-Martin, EM; Sanz-Rodriguez, F; Ramirez, JR; Morales-Angulo, C; Zarrabeitia, R; Perez-Molino, A; Bernabeu, C, y; Botella, LM. Therapeutic action of tranexamic acid in hereditary haemorrhagic telangiectasia (HHT), regulation of ALK-1/endoglin pathway in endothelial cells. *Thromb Haemost*, 2007, 97, 254-62.

[81] Perez-Gomez, E; Eleno, N; Lopez-Novoa, JM; Ramirez, JR; Velasco, B; Letarte, M; Bernabeu, C, y; Quintanilla, M. Characterization of murine S-endoglin isoform and its effects on tumor development. *Oncogene*, 2005, 24, 4450-61.

[82] Wong, VC; Chan, PL; Bernabeu, C; Law, S; Wang, LD; Li, JL; Tsao, SW; Srivastava, G; Lung, ML. Identification of an invasion and tumor

suppressing gene, Endoglin (ENG), silenced by both epigenetic inactivation and allelic loss in esophageal squamous cell carcinoma. *Int J Cancer*, 2008, 123, 2816-2823.

[83] Pérez-Gómez, E; Villa-Morales, M; Santos, J; Fernández-Piqueras, J; Gamallo, C; Dotor, J; Bernabéu, C; Quintanilla, M. A role for endoglin as a suppressor of malignancy during mouse skin carcinogenesis. *Cancer Res*, 2007, 67, 10268-10277.

[84] Hawinkels, LJ; Kuiper, P; Wiercinska, E; Verspaget, HW; Liu, Z; Pardali, E; Sier, CF, y; ten, Dijke, P. Matrix metalloproteinase-14 (MT1-MMP)-mediated endoglin shedding inhibits tumor angiogenesis. *Cancer Res*, 2010, 70, 4141-50.

[85] Ojeda-Fernandez, L; Barrios, L; Rodriguez-Barbero, A; Recio-Poveda, L; Bernabeu, C; Botella, LM. *Clin Chim Acta*, 2010, Apr 2, 411(7-8), 494-9.

[86] Li, X; Yonenaga, Y; Seki, T. Shortened ALK1 regulatory fragment maintains a specific activity in arteries feeding ischemic tissues. *Gene Ther*, 2009, 16, 1034-1041,

[87] Garrido-Martin, EM; Blanco, FJ; Fernandez-L, A; Langa, C; Vary, CP; Lee, UE; Friedman, SL; Botella, LM, y; Bernabeu, C. Characterization of the human Activin-A receptor type II-like kinase 1 (ACVRL1) promoter and its regulation by Sp1. *BMC Mol Biol*, 2010, 11, 51.

[88] Faughnam, ME; Palda, V; Garcia-Tsao, G; et al. International guidelines for the diagnosis and management of hereditary haemorrhagic telangiectasia. *J Med Genet* 2011, 48, 73-87.

[89] Sabba, C; Morelli, GA; Logrono, LA. Treatment of bleeding in hereditary hemorrhagic telangiectasia with aminocaproic acid. *N Eng J Med*, 1994, 330, 1789-90.

[90] Morales, Angulo, C; Pérez, del; Molino, A; Zarrabeitia, R; et al. Treatment of epistaxis in hereditary hemorrhagic telangiectasia (Rendu Osler Weber disease) with tranexamic acid. *Acta Otorrinolaringol Esp*, 2007, 58, 129-32.

[91] Flieger, D; hainke, S; Fischbach, W. Dramatic improvement in hereditary hemorrhagic telangiectasia after treatment with the vascular endothelial growth factor (VEGF) antagonist bevacizumab. *Ann Hematol*, 2006, 85, 631-2.

[92] Simonds, J; Miller, F; mandel, J; Davidson, TH. The effect of bevacizumab (Avastin) treatment on epistaxis in hereditary hemorrhagic telangiectasia. *Laryngoscope*, 2009, 119, 988-92.

[93] Chavan, A; Schumann-Binarsch, S; Luthe, L. Systemic therapy with bevacizumab in patients with HHT. *Vasa*, 2013, 42, 106-10.

[94] Lebrin, F; Srun, S; Raymond, K; et al. Thalidomide stimulates vessel maturation and reduces epistaxis in individuals with hereditary hemorrhagic. *Nat Med*, 2010, 16, 420-8.

[95] Garrido, A; Sayago, M; López, J. Thalidomide in refractory bleeding due to gastrointestinal angiodysplasias. *Rev Esp Enferm Dig*, 2012, 104, 69-71.

[96] McAlister, VC. Regression of cutaneous and gastrointestina telangiectasia with sirolimus and aspirin in a patient with hereditary hemorrhagic telangiectasia. *Ann Intern Med*, 2006, 144, 226-7.

[97] Albiñana, V; Sanz-Rodriguez, F; Recio-Poveda, L; et al. Inmunosuppresor FK506 increases endoglin and activin receptor-like kinase 1 expression and modulates transforming growth factor-β_1 signaling in endothelial cells. *Mol Pharmacol*, 2011, 79, 833-43.

[98] Mager, JJ; Gussem, EM; Disch, FJ; et al. A pilot study on the effect of acetylcisteine on epistaxis and quality of life in HHT. *Hematology Meeting Reports*, 2007, 19.

[99] de, Gussem, EM; Snijder, RJ; Disch, FJ; Zanen, P; Westermann, CJ, y; Mager, JJ. (2009). The effect of N-acetylcysteine on epistaxis and quality of life in patients with HHT, a pilot study. *Rhinology*, 47, 85-8.

[100] Jameson, JJ; Cave, DR. Hormonal and antihormonal therapy for epistaxis in hereditary hemorrhagic telangiectasia. *Laryngoscope*, 2004, 114, 705-9.

[101] Korzenik, JR. Danazol in the treatment of gastrointestinal hemorrhage in HHT. *Gastroenterology*, 1995, 108, 207.

[102] Zacharski, LR; Dunbar, SD; Newsom, WA, Jr. Hemostatic effects of tamoxifen in HHT. *Thrombosis and Haemostasis*, 2001, 85, 371-2.

[103] Yaniv, E; Preis, M; Shevro, J. Anti-estrogen therapy for HHT-a long term clinical trial. *Rhinology*, 2011, 49, 214-6.

[104] Albiñana, V; Bernabeu-Herreo, ME; Zarrabeitia, R; et al. Estrogen therapy for hereditary hemorrhagic telangiectasia (HHT):effects of raloxifen on endoglin and ALK1 expression in endothelial cells. *Thromb Haemost*, 2010, 103, 525-34.

[105] Albiñana, V; Recio-Poveda, L; Zarrabeitia, R; et al. Propranolol as antiangiogenic candidate for the therapy of HHT. *Thromb Haemost* 2012, 108, 41-53

[106] Shovlin, CL; Sulaiman, NL; Govani, FS; et al. Elevated factor VIII in hereditary haemorrhagic telangiectasia (HHT):association with venous thromboembolism. *Thromb Haemost*, 2007, 98, 1031-9.

[107] Pagella, F; Matti, E; Chu, F; et al. Argon plasma coagulation is an effective treatment for HHT patients with severe nosebleeds. *Acta Otolaryngol*, 2013, 133, 174-86.

[108] Karnezis, TT; Davidson, TM. Treatment of hereditary hemorrhagic telangiectasia with submucosal and topical bevacizumab therapy. *Laryngoscope*, 2012, 122, 495-7.

[109] Morais, D; Millás, T; Zarrabeitia, R; et al. Local sclerotherapy with polydocanol (AethoxysKlerol®) for the treatment of epistaxis in Rendu-Osler-Weber or HHT:15 years of experience. *Rhinology*, 2012, 50, 80-6.

[110] Harvey, RJ; Kanagalingan, J; Lund, VJ. The impact of septodermoplasty and potassium-titanyl-phosphate (KTP) laser therapy in the treatment of HHT-related epistaxis. *Am J Rhinol*, 2008, 22, 182-7.

[111] Richer, SL; Geisthoff, VW; Livada, N; et al. The Young´s procedure for severe epistaxis from hereditary hemorrhagic telangiectasia. *Am J Rhinol Allergy*, 2012, 26, 401-4.

[112] Pollak, JS; Saluja, S; Thabet, A; et al. Clinical and anatomic outcomes after embolotherapy of pulmonary arteriovenous malformations. *J Vasc Interv Radiol*, 2006, 17, 35-44.

[113] Lacombe, P; Lagrange, C; Beauchet, A. Diffuse pulmonary arteriovenous malformations in HHT:long-term results of embolization according to the extent of lung involvement. *Chest* 2009, 135, 1031-7

[114] Lee, DW; White, RI; Egglin, TK. Embolotherapy of large pulmonary arteriovenous malformations:long-term results. *Ann Thorac Surg*, 1997, 64, 930-9.

[115] Shovlin, CL; Jackson, JE; Bamford, KB. Primary determinants of ischaemic stroke/brain abscess risks are independent of severity of pulmonary arteriovenous malformations in HHT. *Thorax*, 2008, 63, 259-66.

[116] Shovlin, C; Bamford, K; Wray, D. Post-NICE 2008:Antibiotic prophylaxis prior to dental procedures for patients with pulmonary arteriovenous malformations and hereditary hemorrhagic telangiectasia. *Br Dent J*, 2008, 205, 531-3.

[117] Sopeña, B; Pérez-Rodríguez, MT; Portela, D. High prevalence of pulmonary hypertension in patients with hereditary hemorrhagic telangiectasia. *Eur J Intern Med*, 2013, 24, 30-4.

[118] Buscarini, E; Plauchu, H; Garcia-Tsao, G. Liver involvement in hereditary hemorrhagic telangiectasia:consensus recomendations. *Liver Int*, 2006, 26, 1040-6.

[119] Dupuis-Girod, S; Ginon, I; Saurin, JC. Bevacizumab in patients with hereditary hemorrhagic telangiectasia and severe hepatic vascular malformations and high cardiac output. *JAMA*, 2012, 307, 948-55.

[120] Buscarini, E; Leandro, G; Conte, D; et al. Natural history and outcome of hepatic vascular malformations in a large cohort of patients with hereditary hemorrhagic telangiectasia. *Dig Dis Sci*, 2011, 56, 2166-78.

[121] De, Cillis, E; Burdi, N; Bortone, AS; et al. Endovascular treatment of pulmonary and cerebral arteriovenous malformations in patients affected by HHT. *Curr Pharm Des*, 2006, 12, 1243-8.

[122] Meisel, HJ; Mansmann, U; Alvarez, H; et al. Cerebral arteriovenous malformations and associated aneurysms:analysis of 305 cases from a series of 662 patients. *Neurosurgery*, 2000, 46, 793-800.

[123] Mathis, S; Dupuis-Girod, S; Plauchu, H; et al. Cerebral abscesses in hereditary haemorrhagic telangiectasia:a clinical and microbiological evaluation. *Clin Neurol Neurorurg*, 2012, 114, 235-40.

[124] Swietlik, E; Doboszynska, A. Recurrence of arteriovenous malformations with life-threatening complications in a pregnant women with hereditary hemorrhagic telangiectasia. *J Physiol Pharmacol*, 2008, 59, 683-8.

[125] Goussous, T; Heynes, A; Najarian, K. Hereditary hemorrhagic telangiectasia patient presenting a high cardiac failure during pregnancy. *Cardiol Res Pract*, 2009.

[126] Shovlin, CL; Sodhi, V; McCarthy, A. estimates of maternal risks of pregnancy for women with hereditary hemorrhagic telangiectasia (Osler-Weber-Rendu syndrome):suggested approach for obstetric services. *BJOG*, 2008, 115, 1108-15.

[127] Wain, K; Swanson, K; Watson, W; et al. Hereditary hemorrhagic telangiectasia and risks for adverse pregnancy outcomes. *Am J Med Genet A*, 2012, 2009-14.

[128] Giordano, P; Lenato, GM; Suppresa, P; et al. Hereditary hemorrhagic telangiectasia:arteriovenous malformations in children. *J Pediatr*, 2013, 13.

[129] Mei-Zahav, M; Letarte, M; Faughnanm, ME; et al. Symptomatic children with hereditary hemorrhagic telangiectasia, a pediatric center experience. *Arch Pediatr Adolesc Med*, 2006, 160, 596-601.

In: Autosomal Dominant Disorders   ISBN: 978-1-62808-760-4
Editors: P. Marciano and D. M. Lanza   © 2013 Nova Science Publishers, Inc.

Chapter 3

Osteogenesis Imperfecta

Colin R. Paterson [*]

Formerly Reader in Medicine in the University of Dundee,
Dundee, Scotland, UK

Abstract

Osteogenesis imperfecta is the most common heritable cause of
fractures in children. It is not a single disorder but a large group of
diseases most, but not all, being caused by defects of the genes coding for
collagen. Autosomal dominant inheritance is the most common finding in
familial cases but new mutations occur. Autosomal recessive inheritance
does occur and mosaicism is recognized.

The great molecular heterogeneity is reflected in great clinical and
radiological variation. Some cases are so severe that survival beyond
intra-uterine life is impossible. At the other extreme some patients,
undoubtedly affected their family history, have few fractures and live
normal lives. Fractures often occur spontaneously and previously
asymptomatic fractures in various stages of healing are often found
radiologically. While most symptomatic fractures are diaphyseal, all
types of fractures including metaphyseal fractures, rib fractures and skull
fractures do occur.

Modern management involves good orthopaedic surgery; it is
particularly important to avoid prolonged immobilisation of limbs to

[*] Correspondence: Dr C R Paterson, Temple Oxgates, Longforgan, Dundee DD2 5HS, UK, Tel:
+44 1382 360240, Email:c.s.paterson@btinternet.com.

avoid superimposed osteopenia. Drug therapy, particularly with pamidronate, may be appropriate in children with the more severe forms of the disorder. Specific attention may be needed to scoliosis, basilar invagination or deafness. Good occupational therapy to maximise mobility is important. Children with osteogenesis imperfecta have normal intelligence and good education is vital.

Introduction

Osteogenesis imperfecta (OI) is the most common bone dysplasia causing fractures in childhood. In western countries it has a prevalence of about 1 in 10,000. It occurs in all races.

Classification and Genetics

The most widely used classification of OI based on clinical and radiological features is that of Sillence et al [1]. These authors suggested four major types, each of which has subsequently been subdivided (Table 1). It is important to recognize that there is little relationship between the Sillence type and the underlying mutation. Each Sillence type includes patients with many different mutations. Nevertheless the Sillence classification has been invaluable over the years in allowing consistent reporting of the clinical features of each case.

In recent years a group of clinicians in Montreal has suggested the addition of three further types, V, VI and VII (Table 1). Type V patients were earlier included in type IV but were distinct in having a tendency to form hyperplastic callus after a fracture and calcification of the interosseous membrane of the forearm. These patients were also distinctive in having an IFTM5 mutation [2]. Patients with OI type VI were also clinically similar to type IV patients but had distinctive bone histology with an excess of osteoid. They had a distinctive mutation in SERPINF1 [3]. OI type VII is the name given to an unusual form of severe OI inherited in an autosomal recessive manner found in a small group of indigenous people in northern Quebec [4]. It is not thought to be caused by a mutation in the collagen genes.

Even among patients with the same mutation there is considerable variation in clinical severity [5]. Similarly within a single family the severity of the disorder may vary greatly. The reason for these variations is not known.

One exception is provided by parental mosaicism in which, for example, a clinically normal parent or a mildly affected parent has a severely affected child [6-8]. A further cause for variation within a family occurs when parents who are heterozygous for a mutation and show minor features of OI have a child who is homozygous for the mutation and severely affected [9].

Table 1. Clinical features of the different types of OI in the Sillence scheme together with principal subsequent additions

Type	Features	Genetics
I*	Mild disease usually. Blue or grey sclerae. Normal growth	Autosomal dominant New mutations frequent
II**	Severe disease leading to multiple intrauterine fractures, stillbirth or early neonatal death	Autosomal recessive New mutations
III	Severe disease with fractures at birth and progressive deformity. Often very short stature. Dentinogenesis imperfecta common	Most commonly new mutations of autosomal dominant disorder
IV*	Mild to moderate severity. Normal sclerae except in infancy	Autosomal dominant. New mutations frequent
V	Moderate to severe bone fragility. Hypertrophic callus after fractures. Calcification of interosseous membrane	Autosomal dominant
VI	Moderate to severe bone fragility and deformity. Distinctive bone histology	Autosomal dominant
VII	Moderate to severe disease	Autosomal recessive

* Subdivided: IA and IVA have normal teeth; IB and IVB have dentinogenesis imperfecta.
** Subdivided: A, B and C in relation to the radiological findings.

Biochemical Causes

The mechanical strength of bone depends in part on its content of type I collagen and abnormalities of collagen have been thought since the 1970s to underlie OI [10]. Chemical studies of collagen produced by cultured fibroblasts from patients with OI showed abnormalities. In addition families with dominantly inherited OI had consistent linkage to the two genes coding for type I collagen, COL1A1 and COL1A2 [10, 11].

In 1985 the first mutation was identified, an internal deletion in COL1A1 that had caused a lethal form of OI [12, 13]. By 2007 no less than 832 distinct mutations had been reported [14]. Most of these are private mutations, mutations unique to one individual or family. Deletions are now thought to be an uncommon cause of OI. Exon skipping, due to mutations at splice donor or acceptor sites, is more common. The most common type of mutation by far causes the substitution of a single amino acid.

The structure of a collagen molecule is a triple helix of two alpha 1 chains and one alpha 2 chain. Both contain glycine residues at every third position. These are important structurally; their replacement by bulkier residues distorts the triple helix and prevents the neat packing of molecules into fibrils. Most of the recognized mutations in OI involve substitutions of glycine [15, 16].

The correlation between the nature of the mutation and the clinical features in affected patients is very imperfect. For example substitution of glycine by serine in the alpha 1 chain causes a more severe disease than the same substitution in the alpha 2 chain [5]. In addition a single mutation in apparently unrelated families can result in substantial variation in the clinical phenotype in terms of severity and associated findings [5]. One further cause of clinical variability is somatic mosaicism; an unaffected or mildly affected parent may be associated with a severely affected child [6, 7]. In general blue sclerae are more associated with COL1A1 mutations, particularly those near the amino terminal. Dentinogenesis imperfecta (DI) was most common with mutations in the central region and near the carboxy terminal both in COL1A1 and COL1A2.

It should be noted that mutations in the genes coding for type 1 collagen are not the only causes of OI. It has long been recognized that a minority of patients with OI have no evidence of a mutation in COL1A1 or COL1A2. Some patients have a clearly autosomal recessive inheritance. Many of these disorders are now known to be caused by mutations affecting the proteins involved in the formation of mature collagen.

The formation of collagen is a complex process. The precursors of the alpha 1 and alpha 2 chains are known as procollagens and have peptide chains at both amino- and carboxy-terminals in addition to the future helical portions. These procollagen chains undergo several further steps including the hydroxylation of some proline residues to hydroxyproline with the enzyme prolyl hydroxylase. The procollagen chains come together to give the triple helix and the additional chains at each end are cleaved off. Mutations affecting one of the cleavage sites cause an unusual form of OI with dense bones [17, 18].

Mutations leading to OI, often as a recessive disorder, have now been identified in genes coding for each of the proteins involved in a complex consisting of prolyl 3-hydroxylase, cartilage-associated proteins (CRTAP) and cyclophilin B [19, 20]. Further genes in which mutations have been shown to cause recessively inherited OI include FKBP10, which also causes Bruck syndrome with contractures, and SERPINF 1, which causes OI type VI [3, 21]. OI type V is an autosomal dominant disorder caused by mutations in the gene IFITM5 which codes for a skeletal protein, BRIL, whose function is not yet known [2]. The many mutations that have been shown to underlie OI are recorded in a continuously updated database [22]. Collagen maturation is dependent on the availability of both copper and ascorbic acid. Collagen defects leading to symptoms including fractures are well recognized in copper deficiency and in scurvy.

Clinical Features

While the hallmark of the disorder is the increased tendency to fractures other clinical signs may be present. These include blue or grey sclerae, increased joint laxity, impaired growth, liability to bruising, odd shaped skull, dentinogenesis imperfecta, excessive sweating and premature deafness. Most but not all of these clinical features can be associated with the disorders of collagen which are thought to underlie most cases. Few patients have all these signs and some, undoubtedly affected on the basis of family history, have none.

Fractures

The fractures may occur with little or no recognised trauma or with normal handling. Some asymptomatic fractures may be found when X-rays are taken for other reasons. Fractures usually occur without evidence of any local bruising because little trauma is involved. The increased liability to bruising or petechial haemorrhages is thought to result from the increased fragility of small blood vessels [23]. The paradox that fractures occur with few bruises in a child who also has an increased liability to bruising is shared with other bone disorders that cause fractures [24].

In OI fractures may be unpredictable; there may be long gaps between symptomatic fractures in an individual patient (Figure 1). It should be noted that the fracture rate diminishes in the teenage years in all types of OI. In older men the fracture rate remains low in later life but in women there is an increase in fracture rate, particularly vertebral crush fractures after the menopause (Figure 2) [25].

The fractures of OI may include symptomatic long bone fractures, including transverse, oblique and spiral fractures [26]. Metaphyseal fractures are well recognized and usually asymptomatic (Figure 3).

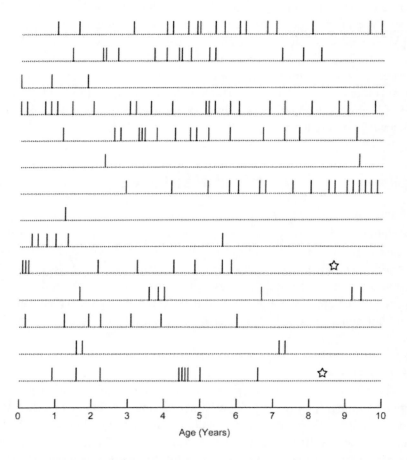

Figure 1. Incidence of fractures in 14 patients with OI type IVA for whom complete records were available for at least eight years. In two cases details were not available for later than the point marked with a star. Data of Paterson et al 1987 [77].

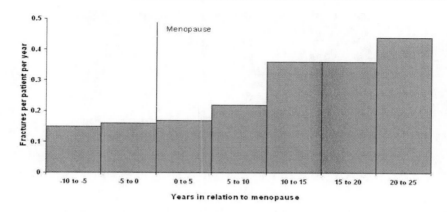

Figure 2. Fractures per patient per year in relation to time of the menopause in 30 women with OI type IA. Data of Paterson et al 1984 [25].

Skull fractures are well-recognized [27]. Rib fractures occur and are usually asymptomatic. That these do occur is illustrated by Figure 4 which shows a child on the day of birth later thought to have OI type III. Multiple rib fractures of different dates are seen; all occurred *in utero*.

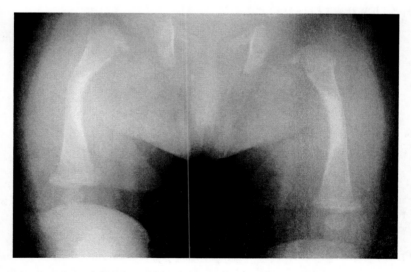

Figure 3. Metaphyseal fractures of both femora in a three day old child later recognized as having OI type IVA.

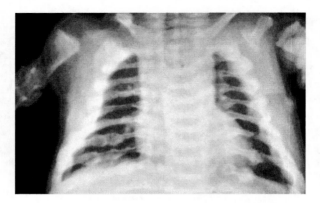

Figure 4. Chest x-ray of a boy on the day of birth showing multiple rib fractures of different ages, all of which had occurred *in utero*. He was later thought to have OI type III.

One specific cause of symptomatic fractures in OI needs to be highlighted. The standard tests for congenital dislocation of the hip are those of Ortolani and of Barlow. Carrying out such tests in infants with OI, or whose family history implies that they may have OI, is not advisable; fractures of the femur may occur (Figure 5) [28].

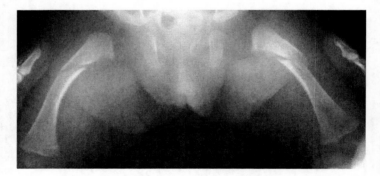

Figure 5. Bilateral femoral fractures found after an examination for congenital hip dislocation in an infant girl with a family history of OI type IVB.

Dental Abnormalities

Dentine also contains collagen and a substantial proportion of OI patients have overt dentinogenesis imperfecta (DI). The teeth are discoloured, translucent and fragile. The severity varies greatly among OI patients. Detailed study of the teeth, including scanning electron microscopy, has shown that all OI patients have abnormalities in the teeth [29]. It should be noted that DI can exist without OI; this disorder is known as DI type II [30]. It is also inherited as an autosomal dominant.

Sclerae

The grey or blue sclerae are among the best known features of OI. They are present in about two thirds of patients and play a part in the conventional classification. The scleral discolouration is thought to reflect thinness of scleral collagen so that the underlying pigment shows through. The assessment of scleral colour is not an exact science; attempts to quantify it using a paint colour strip have not been widely used. Also it should be noted that some blue colouration is seen in normal infants.

Premature Deafness

Hearing loss can occur in all types of OI. Most of the patients who develop hearing loss have their first symptom before the age of 40 but a few have a later age of onset (Table 2) [31, 32].

Table 3 shows the likelihood of developing deafness in each type of OI. Most surveys have shown that the deafness associated with OI has no single cause. Most patients have a mixed pattern; smaller numbers have sensorineural or conductive patterns [32, 33].

Table 2. Age of onset of hearing impairment in 77 patients out of 133 OI patients aged 17 or more [32]

Age range	Number of patients
0-10	1
10-20	19
20-30	27
30-40	12
40-50	10
50-60	4
60-70	2
70-80	1
80-90	1

Table 3. Proportion of OI patients of each type who had symptoms of hearing impairment at age 30 [31]

Sillence type	Number of patients aged 30 or more	Number of patients with hearing impairment at age 30	Percentage affected at age 30
IA	276	90	33
IB	60	18	30
III	23	12	52
IVA	32	3	9
IVB	52	15	29
Uncertain	18	7	39

Cardiovascular Problems

Hypertension appears to be common in adults with OI [34]. Valvular heart disorders, particularly aortic and mitral regurgitation, are also found and often require surgery [34, 35].

Excessive Sweating

Excessive sweating has long been recognized as a symptom in children with OI but no explanation can be made from collagen biochemistry. A postoperative febrile response is more common in children with OI than in normal controls but appears to be harmless [36].

Joint Laxity

Increased laxity of joints is seen in a substantial minority of patients with OI. It may lead to confusion with the Ehlers-Danlos syndrome, some forms of which also result from mutations in the genes coding for collagen. Joint laxity may contribute to the disability resulting from OI, for example in permitting hyperextension of the fingers or in causing instability of the ankles.

Neurological Problems

Basilar invagination is an uncommon but very serious complication of OI and some other bone disorders. It consists of the upward displacement of parts of the occipital bone surrounding the foramen magnum leading to pressure from the upper cervical spine on the brainstem. Symptoms include headache in the neck and occiput, often worse with coughing, sneezing or straining, trigeminal neuralgia, giddiness, weakness in the arms or legs and bladder disorders [37]. Among the physical signs are nystagmus, facial spasm, nerve paresis, proprioceptive defects, pyramidal tract signs and papilloedema [37]. The change in the skull shape may lead to changes in the face including recession of the maxilla and prominence of the mandible (prognathism). While basilar invagination occurs in all types of OI, basilar invagination with neurological consequences is most common in OI type IV B [37].

Intracranial haemorrhage may occur in OI [38, 39] and is a significant cause of death [40].

Impaired Growth

Post-natal growth is normal in many cases of OI type I, reduced in most type IV cases and substantially reduced in OI type III. There is no evidence of growth hormone deficiency [41, 42].

Temperament

One striking feature of many OI patients is their generally positive approach to life often despite appreciable disabilities. This has been confirmed formally [43, 44]. Educational achievements are usually normal despite disabilities [43].

Life Expectancy

Life expectancy is normal in OI type IA, marginally reduced in OI types IB, IVA and IVB, and appreciably reduced in OI type III [45]. Most patients with type I and type IV forms of OI have a normal lifespan and die of causes unrelated to their OI. In many type III patients premature deaths are caused, particularly in childhood, by respiratory problems resulting from kyphoscoliosis. OI plays a direct part in deaths due to basilar invagination and intracranial haemorrhage.

Radiology and Densitometry

The wide range of clinical severity in OI is reflected in a wide range of radiological appearances. Patients with OI types II and III usually have obvious abnormalities from and often before the time of birth. These include fractures which have occurred *in utero* (Figure 4). Most patients with type I and type IV OI have radiologically normal bone at birth. Radiological appearances often remain normal throughout life in bones which have not sustained fractures.

One radiological sign may be helpful in diagnosis. Wormian bones are additional bones, usually in the occipital part of the skull, completely surrounded by a suture line. Conventionally more than 10 such bones are regarded as significant for the diagnosis of OI. In a recent study significant numbers of Wormian bones were seen in 35 percent of patients with OI type I, in 78 percent of patients with OI type IV and in 96 percent of patients with OI type III [46]. It is important to note that excessive numbers of Wormian bones may be found in other disorders including cretinism, cleido-cranial dysostosis and Menkes syndrome [47].

Densitometry

Attempts to assess bone density from ordinary X-rays are imprecise and should not be used [48]. It is inappropriate to comment that a "normal" appearance on ordinary X-rays excludes OI or any other bone disease. However it is true that a substantial number of OI patients have low values when formal densitometry is undertaken.

In our experience of adults with OI (for whom we had a well established reference range) most patients were below the mean for the reference group but many had a higher bone density than the lower reference limit (minus 2 standard deviations) [49]. Similar findings were obtained with DXA of the spine [50, 51]. In one study [51] the authors commented that in "some mildly affected patients brittleness may exist with only small reductions in bone mineral content."

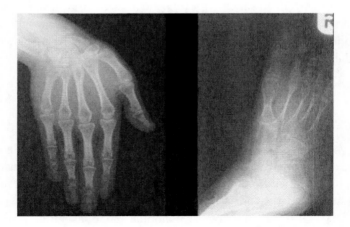

Figure 6. Hand and foot of a young woman with OI type IVB. The hand (left) shows normal appearances while the foot appears severely abnormal. During her childhood and adolescence she had had multiple fractures in the legs.

In children there are only small studies and none of the reference ranges used were satisfactory [52-54]. However it is likely that, as in adults, children with OI have lower bone densities compared with controls but with an appreciable overlap. One difficulty in this field is the continuing lack of robust reference ranges appropriate for the densitometers used.

One further difficulty affecting both adults and children is that a fracture with a period of immobilisation may itself lead to diminished bone density of the limb concerned. This may lead to false assumptions about bone density in the underlying condition. This problem is illustrated in Figure 6.

Clinical Biochemistry

Routine investigations such as serum calcium, inorganic phosphate and alkaline phosphatase usually show no abnormality in OI. One exception is that serum alkaline phosphatase may rise if there are multiple healing fractures. It is important to note that normal findings in these tests do not exclude OI.

A number of other biochemical abnormalities have been found in some patients with OI. These include a high urine calcium [55], a high urinary excretion of cross-linked collagen peptides [56] and low serum levels of carboxy-terminal propeptides of human type I procollagen (PICP) [57, 58]. None of these investigations has been evaluated as a test for OI.

One recent study suggested that some children with OI may also be deficient in vitamin D [59]. The actual levels were not given but it seems likely that children with any disability are at risk of spending less time exposed to sunshine than their peers.

Biochemical investigations used for the diagnosis of OI are of two main types. Some examine the chemistry of the collagen from cultured fibroblasts derived from skin biopsies [60]. Others search for mutations in the genes coding for type I collagen. These tests are useful in the confirmation of OI in cases in which it is not clinically obvious. However there is no information on the likelihood of finding abnormalities in a large unselected group of OI patients. As a result we have little information on the frequency of false negatives. Table 4 shows the findings in two studies; they indicate that in both false negatives are most likely in patients in whom the clinical findings are least helpful. It is not correct to say that a negative result excludes OI.

Table 4. Percentage of positive findings in known cases of osteogenesis imperfecta investigated by collagen analysis and by mutation detection

OI type	Collagen analysis	Mutation detection
Type I	94%	94%
Type III	84%	81%
Type IV	84%	69%
Type unknown	50%	

Collagen analysis data of Wenstrup et al [76]. Mutation detection data in personal communication from Dr D Prockop May 2000

Differential Diagnoses

In the past numerous cases of OI have initially been diagnosed as child abuse [61-64]. Children with OI may have fractures that the parents or carers cannot explain (Figure 7). They may then be found to have other fractures not clinically suspected; they may have multiple fractures of different ages. The bones may otherwise appear to be normal on ordinary X-rays. It is not surprising therefore that cases of misdiagnosis occur. However it is likely that a substantially larger number of cases of misdiagnosis result from other bone disorders which also mimic accepted descriptions of abuse [24]. These include the osteopathy of prematurity and vitamin D deficiency rickets.

Management

It is likely that occupational therapists, physiotherapists and orthopaedic surgeons have more to contribute to the management of these patients than any drug therapy but it is important to review the current position.

Drug Therapy

Many drugs have been tried in OI including calcium, anabolic steroids, vitamin C, calcitonin and fluoride. None of these has been shown to be of value in properly controlled trials. The practical difficulties in mounting such trials in OI are substantial because of the variable natural history..

Short stature is a common feature of OI and several trials of growth hormone have been undertaken [65]. While growth velocity increased in the treated group the differences were small and there was no evidence that the final height would be improved. There is no evidence that growth hormone deficiency plays any part in the short stature of OI.

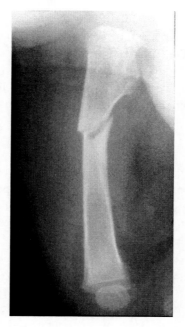

Figure 7. Fracture of left femur in a boy of four months, one of twins. Since the bone appeared normal radiologically it was assumed that considerable force was involved and a care order was sought for both boys. However it later became clear that his father, uncle and grandfather all had pale blue sclerae, dentinogenesis imperfecta and a typical history of OI. By the time of the hearing the boy and his twin brother had obvious dentinogenesis imperfecta.

Numerous trials have been undertaken in recent years of various bisphosphonates including alendronate, neridronate, olpadronate, risdronate and zoledronic acid. By far the greatest number of studies have involved pamidronate usually by cyclic intravenous infusions [66, 67]. All the studies found that bone turnover decreased and bone mineral density increased. Many studies have reported a decrease in the number of fractures in the more severe types of OI. However, in some of these the comparison was only with pre-treatment fracture rates; it should be remembered that the fracture rate in untreated OI is extremely variable, often decreasing with age.

The underlying premise in many of these studies is that a rise in bone density is in itself a good thing. However it should be recognised that bisphosphonate treatment in anyone will decrease bone turnover and increase bone density. Decreased bone remodelling may have long term disadvantages for fracture risk. At present it seems that cyclic bisphosphonate therapy is probably advantageous for children with the more severe types of OI but not for adults or for children with milder forms of OI.

One report described clinical responses to bone marrow transplantation in children with severe OI [68]. While initial results were encouraging this strategy does not appear to have been pursued since.

In postmenopausal women with OI the case for low-dose hormone replacement therapy probably outweighs the case against.

Pain Relief

In children, as in adults, pain relief is important after fractures. Paracetamol is effective in mild to moderate pain. For more severe pain non-steroidal anti-inflammatory drugs may be helpful as are opioids.

Orthopaedic Surgery

Good orthopaedic care is needed for fractures to avoid deformity, and therefore increased risk of subsequent fractures. However the period of immobilisation should be minimised to reduce the risk of superimposed disuse osteoporosis. Various forms of intramedullary fixation including telescopic rods can be used in children with recurrent fractures [69].

Scoliosis is common in OI. The conventional view is that if the scoliosis does not exceed 45° conservative management is appropriate. Bracing is ineffective. If the scoliosis exceeds 45° it is thought that posterior spinal fusion is justifiable. However surgery is often difficult because of bleeding and the innate fragility of the bone. Newer techniques appear to be effective [70].

Surgery for Basilar Invagination

Basilar invagination with neurological complications is treated surgically by a transoral clivectomy. This not only halts disease progression in most patients but also provides a sustainable long-term functional outcome [71, 72].

Deafness

As with deafness in general the first step involves the use of hearing aids. In OI, particularly with conductive deafness, stapes surgery usually has good long-term results [73, 74]. In appropriate cases cochlear implantation is a safe and feasible procedure [75].

Dental Care

Good dental care is important in OI, particularly in patients with overt dentinogenesis imperfecta. The teeth in this condition are not only discoloured but fragile. Veneers may be useful for cosmetic reasons but do not contribute to strength.

Some cola drinks are particularly undesirable because of their acidity. Supplemental fluoride may be desirable.

Education

Despite the disadvantage of repeated hospital admissions children with OI do well in education; many have above average potential [43]. A good education is of vital importance for the future. In general, mainstream education is usually preferable to schools for the disabled.

Acknowledgments

I am grateful to Dr. Elspeth Paterson for her careful review of this paper in draft, and to Mr Jake McLaughlin and Ms Kirsteen Bovill for excellent secretarial assistance.

References

[1]   Sillence DO, Senn A, Danks DM. Genetic heterogeneity in osteogenesis imperfecta. *J. Med. Genet.* 1979;16: 101-16.

[2]   Rauch F, Moffat P, Cheung M et al. Osteogenesis imperfecta type V: marked phenotypic variability despite the presence of the IFITM5 c. 14C>T mutation in all patients. *J. Med. Genet.* 2013;50: 21-4.

[3]   Homan EP, Rauch F, Grafe I et al. Mutations in SERPINF1 cause osteogenesis imperfecta type VI. *J. Bone Miner. Res.* 2011;26: 2798-803.

[4]   Ward LM, Rauch F, Travers R et al. Osteogenesis imperfecta type VII: an autosomal recessive form of brittle bone disease. *Bone* 2002;31: 12-8.

[5]   Rauch F, Lalic L, Roughley P, Glorieux FH. Genotype-phenotype correlations in nonlethal osteogenesis imperfecta caused by mutations in the helical domain of collagen type I. *Eur. J. Med. Genet.* 2010;18: 642-7.

[6]   Cohen-Solal L, Zolezzi F, Pignatti PF, Mottes M. Intrafamilial variable expressivity of osteogenesis imperfecta due to mosaicism for a lethal G382R substitution in the COL1A1 gene. *Mol. Cell. Probes.* 1996;10: 219-25.

[7]   Lund AM, Nicholls AC, Schwartz M, Skovby F. Parental mosaicism and autosomal dominant mutations causing structural abnormalities of collagen I are frequent in families with osteogenesis imperfecta type III/IV. *Acta Paediatr.* 1997;86: 711-8.

[8]   Pyott SM, Pepin MG, Schwarze U, Yang K, Smith G, Byers PH. Recurrence of perinatal lethal osteogenesis imperfecta in sibships: parsing the risk between parental mosaicism for dominant mutations and autosomal recessive inheritance. *Genet. Med.* 2011;13: 125-30.

[9]   De Paepe A, Nuytinck L, Raes M, Fryns J. Homozygosity by descent for a COL1A2 mutation in two sibs with severe osteogenesis imperfecta and mild clinical expression in the heterozygotes. *Hum. Genet.* 1997;99: 478-83.

[10] Sykes B, Ogilvie D, Wordsworth P et al. Consistent linkage of dominantly inherited osteogenesis imperfecta to the type I collagen loci: COL1A1 and COL1A2. *Am. J. Hum. Genet.* 1990;46: 293-307.

[11] Mottes M, Cugola L, Cappello N, Pignatti PF. Segregation analysis of dominant osteogenesis imperfecta in Italy. *J. Med. Genet.* 1990;27: 367-70.

[12] Chu ML, Gargiulo V, Williams CJ, Ramirez F. Multiexon deletion in an osteogenesis imperfecta variant with increased type III collagen mRNA. *J. Biol. Chem.* 1985;260: 691-4.

[13] Barsh GS, Roush CL, Bonadio J, Byers PH, Gelinas RE. Intron-mediated recombination may cause a deletion in an α1 type I collagen

chain in a lethal form of osteogenesis imperfecta. *Proc. Nat. Acad. Sci. USA* 1985;82: 2870-4.

[14] Marini JC, Forlino A, Cabral WA et al. Consortium for osteogenesis imperfecta mutations in the helical domain of type I collagen: regions rich in lethal mutations align with collagen binding sites for integrins and proteoglycans. *Hum. Mutat.* 2007;28: 209-21.

[15] Roughley PJ, Rauch F, Glorieux FH. Osteogenesis imperfecta – clinical and molecular diversity. *Eur. Cell. Mater.* 2003;5: 41-7.

[16] Forlino A, Cabral WA, Barnes AM, Marini JC. New perspectives on osteogenesis imperfecta. *Nature Rev. Endocr.* 2011;7: 540-57.

[17] Lindahl K, Barnes AM, Fratzl-Zelman N et al. COL1 C-propeptide cleavage site mutations cause high bone mass osteogenesis imperfecta. *Hum. Mutat.* 2011;32: 598-609.

[18] Takagi M, Hori N, Chinen Y et al. Heterozygous C-propeptide mutations in COL1A1: osteogenesis imperfecta type IIC and dense bone variant. *Am. J. Med. Gene A* 2011;155A: 2269-73.

[19] Morello R, Bertin TK, Chen Y et al. CRTAP is required for prolyl 3-hydroxylation and mutations cause recessive osteogenesis imperfecta. *Cell* 2006;127: 291-304.

[20] Van Dijk FS, Nesbitt IM, Zwikstra EH et al. PPIB mutations cause severe osteogenesis imperfecta. *Am. J. Hum. Genet.* 2009;85: 521-7.

[21] Kelley BP, Malfait F, Bonafe L et al. Mutations in FKBP10 cause recessive osteogenesis imperfecta and Bruck syndrome. *J. Bone Miner. Res.* 2010;26: 666-72.

[22] Dalgleish RA Database of osteogenesis imperfecta and Ehlers-Danlos syndrome variants. www.le.ac.uk/ge/collagen

[23] Evensen SA, Myhre L, Stormorken H. Haemostatic studies in osteogenesis imperfecta. *Scand. J. Haematol.* 1984;33: 177-9.

[24] Paterson CR. Bone disease and fractures in early childhood. In: Turner RA, Rogers HO, eds *Child Abuse.* New York: Nova, 2012 pp #27-52.

[25] Paterson CR, McAllion S, Stellman JL. Osteogenesis imperfecta after the menopause. *N. Engl. J. Med.* 1984;310: 1694-6.

[26] Dent JA, Paterson CR. Fractures in early childhood: osteogenesis imperfecta or child abuse? *J. Pediatr. Orthop.* 1991;11: 184-6.

[27] Charnas LR, Marini JC. Communicating hydrocephalus, basilar invagination, and other neurological features in osteogenesis imperfecta. *Neurology* 1993; 43: 2603-8.

[28] Paterson CR, Beal RJ, Dent JA. Osteogenesis imperfecta: fractures of the femur when testing for congenital dislocation of the hip. *BMJ* 1992;305: 464-6.

[29] Hall RK, Maniere MC, Palamara J, Hemmerle J. Odontoblast dysfunction in osteogenesis imperfecta: an LM, SEM, and ultrastructural study. *Connect Tissue Res.* 2002;43: 401-5.

[30] Malmgren B, Lindskog S, Elgadi A, Norgren S. Clinical , histopathologic, and genetic investigation in two large families with dentinogenesis imperfecta type II. *Hum. Genet.* 2004;114: 491-8.

[31] Paterson CR, Monk EA, McAllion SJ. How common is hearing impairment in osteogenesis imperfecta? *J. Laryngol. Otol.* 2001; 115: 280-2.

[32] Kuurila K, Kaitila I, Johansson R, Grénman R. Hearing loss in Finnish adult patients with osteogenesis imperfecta, a nationwide survey. *Ann. Otol. Rhinol. Laryngol.* 2002;111:939-46.

[33] Pillion JP, Shapiro J. Audiological findings in osteogenesis imperfecta. *J. Am. Acad. Audiol.* 2008;19:595-601.

[34] Radunovic Z, Wekre LL, Diep LM, Steine K. Cardiovascular abnormalities in adults with osteogenesis imperfecta. *Am. Heart J.* 2011;161: 523-9.

[35] Wong RS, Follis FM, Shively BK, Wernly JA. Osteogenesis imperfecta and cardiovascular diseases. *Ann. Thorac. Surg.* 1995;60: 1439-43.

[36] Ghert M, Allen B, Davids J, Stasikelis P, Nicholas D. Increased postoperative febrile response in children with osteogenesis imperfecta. *J. Pediatr. Orthop.* 2003;23: 261-4.

[37] Sillence DO, Craniocervical abnormalities in osteogenesis imperfecta: genetic and molecular correlation. *Pediatr. Radiol.* 1994;24: 427-30.

[38] Sasaki-Adams D, Kulkarni A, Rutka J, Dirks P, Taylor M, Drake JM. Neurosurgical implications of osteogenesis imperfecta in children. *J. Neurosurg. Pediatrics* 2008;1: 229-36.

[39] Faqeih E, Roughley P, Glorieux FH, Rauch F. Osteogenesis imperfecta type III with intracranial hemorrhage and brachydactyly associated with mutations in exon 49 of COL1A2. *Am. J. Med. Genet. A.* 2009;149A: 461-5.

[40] McAllion SJ, Paterson CR. Causes of death in osteogenesis imperfecta. *J. Clin. Path.* 1996;49: 627-30.

[41] Vetter U, Pontz B, Zauner E, Brenner RE, Spranger J. Osteogenesis imperfecta: a clinical study of the first ten years of life. *Calcif Tissue Int* 1992;50: 36-41.

[42] Lund AM, Muller J, Skovby F. Anthropometry of patients with osteogenesis imperfecta. *Arch. Dis. Child* 1999;80: 524-8.

[43] Widmann RF, Laplaza FJ, Bitan FD, Brooks CE, Root L. Quality of life in osteogenesis imperfecta. *Int. Orthop.* 2002;26: 3-6.

[44] Suskauer SJ, Cintas HL, Marini JC, Gerber LH. Temperament and physical performance in children with osteogenesis imperfecta. *Pediatrics* 2003;111: E153-61.

[45] Paterson CR, Ogston SA, Henry RM. Life expectancy in osteogenesis imperfecta. *BMJ* 1996;312: 351.

[46] Semler O, Cheung MS, Glorieux FH, Rauch F. Wormian bones in osteogenesis imperfecta: correlation to clinical findings and genotype. *Am. J. Med. Genet. A* 2010;152A:1681-7.

[47] Cremin B, Goodman H, Spranger J, Beighton P. Wormian bones in osteogenesis imperfecta and other disorders. *Skeletal Radiol.* 1982;8: 35-8.

[48] Williamson MR, Boyd CM, Williamson SL. Osteoporosis: diagnosis by plain chest film versus dual photon bone densitometry. *Skeletal Radiol.* 1990;19: 27-30.

[49] Paterson CR, Mole PA. Bone density in osteogenesis imperfecta may well be normal. *Posgrad. Med. J.* 1994;70: 104-7.

[50] Deodhar AA, Woolf AD. Bone density measurement in osteogenesis imperfecta may well be important. *Postgrad. Med. J.* 1994;70: 463-4.

[51] Lund AM, Mølgaard C, Müller J, Skovby F. Bone mineral content and collagen defects in osteogenesis imperfecta. *Acta Paediatr.* 1999;88: 1083-8.

[52] Zionts LE, Nash JP, Rude R, Ross T, Stott NS. Bone mineral density in children with mild osteogenesis imperfecta. *J. Bone Joint Surg. (Br)* 1995;77-B:143-7.

[53] Moore MS, Minch CM, Kruse RW, Harcke HT, Jacobson L, Taylor A. The role of dual energy x-ray absorptiometry in aiding the diagnosis of pediatric osteogenesis imperfecta. *Am. J. Orthop.* 1998;27: 797-801.

[54] Kutilek S, Bayer M. Quantitative ultrasonometry of the calcaneus in children with osteogenesis imperfecta. *J. Paediatr. Child Health* 2010;46: 592-4.

[55] Chines A, Boniface A, McAlister W, Whyte M. Hypercalciuria in osteogenesis imperfecta: a follow-up study to assess renal effects. *Bone* 1995;16: 333-9.

[56] Brenner RE, Vetter U, Bollen A, Mörike M, Eyre DR. Bone resorption assessed by immunoassay of urinary cross-linked collagen peptides in

patients with osteogenesis imperfecta. *J. Bone Miner. Res.* 1994;9: 993-7.

[57]   Minisola S, Piccioni AL, Rosso R et al. Reduced serum levels of carboxy-terminal propeptide of human type I procollagen in a family with type I-A osteogenesis imperfecta. *Metabolism* 1994;43: 1261-5.

[58]   Prószyńska K, Wieczorek E, Olszaniecka M, Lorenc RS. Collagen peptides in osteogenesis imperfecta, idiopathic juvenile osteoporosis and Ehlers-Danlos syndrome. *Acta Paediatr.* 1996;85: 688-91.

[59]   Kadhim M, Bober MB, Holmes L et al. Vitamin D status in pediatric patients with osteogenesis imperfecta. *Pediatr. Therapeut.* 2011;1:103.

[60]   Marlowe A, Pepin MG, Byers PH. Testing for osteogenesis imperfecta in cases of suspected non-accidental injury. *J. Med. Genet.* 2002;39: 382-6.

[61]   Pandya NK, Baldwin K, Kamath AF, Wenger DR, Hosalkar HS. Unexplained fractures: child abuse or bone disease. *Clin. Orthop. Relat. Res.* 2011;469: 805-12.

[62]   Kocher MS, Dichtel L. Osteogenesis imperfecta misdiagnosed as child abuse. *J. Pediatr. Orthop. B* 2011;20: 440-3.

[63]   D'Eufemia P, Palombaro M, Lodato V et al. Child abuse and osteogenesis imperfecta: how can they still be misdiagnosed? A case report. *Clin. Cases Miner. Bon. Metab.* 2012;9:195-7.

[64]   Haile JT, Carroll VG, Steele RW. Leg pain in an infant. *Clin. Pediatr.* 2010;49:78-81.

[65]   Antoniazzi F, Bertoldo F, Mottes M et al. Growth hormone treatment in osteogenesis imperfecta with quantitative defect of type I collage synthesis. *J. Pediatr.* 1996;129:432-9.

[66]   Astrŏm E, Jorulf H, Sŏderhäll S. Intravenous pamidronate treatment of infants with severe osteogenesis imperfecta. *Arch. Dis. Child* 2007;92:332-8.

[67]   Glorieux FH. Experience with bisphosphonates in osteogenesis imperfecta. *Pediatrics* 2007;119:S163-5.

[68]   Horwitz EM, Prockop DJ, Gordon PL et al. Clinical responses to bone marrow transplantation in children with severe osteogenesis imperfecta. *Blood* 2001;97:1227-31.

[69]   Esposito P, Plotkin H. Surgical treatment of osteogenesis imperfecta: current concepts. *Curr. Opin. Pediatr.* 2008;20:52-7.

[70]   Yilmaz G, Hwang S, Oto M et al. Surgical treatment of scoliosis osteogenesis imperfecta with cement augmented pedicle screw

instrumentation. *J. Spinal. Disord. Tech.* 2012:doi:10.1097/ BSD.obo13e3182624b76.

[71] Hayes M, Parker G, Ell J, Sillence D. Basilar impression complicating osteogenesis imperfecta type IV: the clinical and neuroradiological findings in four cases. *J. Neurol. Neurosurg. Psychiatry* 1999;66:357-64.

[72] Ibrahim AG, Crockard HA. Basilar impression and osteogenesis imperfecta: a 21 year retrospective review of outcomes in 20 patients. *J. Neurosurg. Spine* 2007;7:594-600.

[73] Hultcrantz M, Sääf M. Stapes surgery in osteogenesis imperfecta: a clinical study of 16 patients. *Adv. Otorhinolaryngol.* 2007;65:222-5.

[74] Denoyelle F, Daval M, Leboulanger N et al. Stapedectomy in children: causes and surgical results in 35 cases. *Arch. Otolaryngol. Head Neck. Surg.* 2010;136:1005-8.

[75] Rotteveel LJ, Beynon AJ, Mens LH et al. Cochlear implantation in 3 patients with osteogenesis imperfecta: imaging, surgery and programming issues. *Audiol. Neurootol.* 2008;13:73-85.

[76] Wenstrup RJ, Willing MC, Starman BJ, Byers PH. Distinct biochemical phenotypes predict clinical severity in non lethal variants of osteogenesis imperfecta. *Am. J. Hum. Genet.* 1990;46:975-82.

[77] Paterson CR, McAllion SJ, Shaw JW. Clinical and radiological features of osteogenesis imperfecta type IVA. *Acta Paediatr. Scand.* 1987;44:187-9.

In: Autosomal Dominant Disorders   ISBN: 978-1-62808-760-4
Editors: P. Marciano and D. M. Lanza © 2013 Nova Science Publishers, Inc.

Chapter 4

Autosomal Dominant Disorders Associated to Breast Cancer

Nelly Margarita Macías-Gómez[*]

Laboratorio de Genética Humana; Departamento de Salud y Bienestar.
Centro Universitario del Sur. Ciudad Guzmán, Jalisco, México

Abstract

The sudden rise of new biochemical and molecular techniques, have
enabled a better understanding of the physiological and biochemical
bases of the tumorogenesis, leaving clear that cancer is a "*genetic
condition*". Breast cancer is one of the most common cancers in women,
affecting one in six women among 40-59 years in the world; so it has
been widely studied. Unlike the majority of genetic diseases, in which the
presence of a mutation in a particular gene is sufficient for delineation of
a phenotype (monogenic); in breast cancer, the simple presence of a
mutation in a particular gene is not enough to explain it. Approximately
90% of breast cancer cases occur sporadically and the majority of cases
are caused by mutations in the *BRCA1* or *BRCA2* gene. However, in 5-
10% of cases of breast cancer has been identify an autosomal dominant
transmission, as well as mutations in specific genes such as *TP53, PTEN,
CHECK2 STK11* among others, that considerably increase the
susceptibility to this condition. Autosomal dominant transmission of this
disease has opened a new chapter in cancer medicine since the presence

---

[*] Nellymacias_2000@yahoo.com.mx.

of any of these mutations in a patient, forces the doctor to carry out a deep investigation of the condition in order to establish a prognosis, as well as effective strategies for survival and family prevention. This chapter makes a brief revision of the autosomal dominat disorders Li-Fraumani syndrome, Cowden Disease and Peutz-Jeghers syndrome, which have a high susceptibility to development of breast cancer.

Breast Cancer

The sudden boom of biochemical and molecular techniques, have enabled us to a better understanding of the physiological and biochemical bases of the tumorigenesis, leaving clear that cancer is a genetic "condition". Breast cancer is a disease in which the different cells from breast gain the ability to grow, multiply and become immortal. Is the most common cancers in humans, so it has been widely studied; however, until now there are many questions about the mechanisms involved in their development where several factors as hormonal, reproductive, life style and inheritance play an important role. Even breast cancer mortality has declined in the last 10-15 years (2.3% per year) due to the innovation of diagnostic techniques and more effective treatments, still is a health problem in reproductive women because each year is reported an incidence of 1 million cases, representing 200,000 cases in the EU (27% of all cancers in female) and 320,000 cases in Europe (31% of all cancers in female) (Neville, 2001, Dumitrescu, 2005). In women from United States, breast cancer is the first cancer which represents 22-32% of all types of cancer, as well as being the second cause of death followed by lung cancer (Thull, 2004, Garber, 2005). According with Glocbocan in 2008 was reported 1´384, 155 new cases of breast cancer, which represent the 22.9% of all types of cancer and a mortality of 458,503 (13.7%) (http://globocan.iarc.fr/). Is estimated that a woman who lives 85 years, has one to nine chance of developing breast cancer, however, this risk is not homogeneous for the entire population, since while some women never develop breast cancer, the risk is increased for others. Epidemiological studies in different populations, have been the identification of well established factors that increase or decrease the risk for developing cancer of the breast, as well as other factors that is necessary to conduct more studies in order to identify their contribution (table 1) (Dumitrescu, 2005, Singletary, 2003).

Table 1. Risk factors to Breast Cancer

Biological and geogaphic	Age
	Gender
	Geographic localization
	Race/ Ethnicity
	Hormonal/ Reproductive
Life Style	Alcohol/ Folates
	Diet
	Obesity
	Physical activity
Genetics	Familiar History
	Syndrome associated to Breast Cancer development
Others	Endometriosis
	Tabacco
	Breast density
	Bening breast lesion
	Radiation exposure
	Bone density
	Intake of aspirin and INES

Among the genetics risk factors has been well known, that the affectation of a family member with breast cancer is a strong risk factor, and this risk is estimated depending on the type of cancer, degree of relationship (first or second degree), age at which the family developed the cancer and the number of relatives affected in the family. In this regards, has been estimated that a women with a familiar history in first degree with breast cancer at 50 years or over, have a increase relative risk (RR) of 1.8 and who develop before at 50 years it´s RR is 3.3. Similarly, when there is a history of two affected relatives in the first degree, the RR increases to 3.6 and, 3.9 when affected relatives are more than two (Dumitrescu, 2005, Glover, 2006, Antoniou, 2006). Although approximately 10-20% of breast cancer cases are attributed to hereditary factors, only 5-10% of patients has been identified a specific mutation in high penetrant genes that are transmitted in autosomal dominant manner, and the most widely identified are *Breast Cancer 1* (*BRCA1*) and *Breast Cancer 2* (*BRCA2*). Recently, had been delineated a group of syndromes autosomal dominant that share the susceptibility to develop several types of cancer, including breast cancer: the Li-fraumeni syndrome which has mutations in the

TP53 gene (*Tumor protein 53*), Cowden syndrome with mutations in *PTEN* gene (*Phosphatase and tension homolog*) and Petz-Jeghers with mutation in *STK11* gene (*Serine / threonine kinase 11*) (Dumitrescu, 2005).

Li-Fraumeni Syndrome

Li-Fraumeni syndrome (*LFS*) (MIM-#151623), described for the first time in 1969, is a heterogeneous condition autosomal dominant, with high penetrance. LFS is characterized by the appearance of different types of cancer during the childhood of an individual, as well as several members of the family. The life time risk for cancer develops in patient with LFS is of 73% in males and nearly 100% in females, with the high risk of breast cancer accounting for the difference. Additionally, is important to consider the age of patient, due to the specific risk for males is 19% before to 15 years, 27% between 16-45 years and 54% in older than 45 years. The risk for females is 12 before 15 years, 82% between 16-45 years and 100% in older than 45 years (Malkin, 2011; Evans, 1997). Has been described that LFS family member diagnosed with cancer has a 15% to develop a second cancer, 4% develop a third cancer and 2% has a fourth cancer (Hisada, 1998; Mai, 2012). One of the main types of cancer who develop LFS patients is breast, which is of early presentation (< 40 years) and usually bilateral. LFS is responsible for approximately 1% of familiar breast cancer syndrome. The median age of diagnosis of first malignancy is 25 and approximately 50% of LFS-associated malignancies occur by age 30 years. The median age of onset of breast cancer diagnosis in carriers is about 33 years and no occurred after age 50 years. Overall, woman with LFS has a breast cancer risk of 56% by age 45 and greater than 90% by age 60, with a majority of the cancers occurring under age 40. If the LFS is done, the NCCN guideline suggest the patient being monthly breast self-examinations at age 18, biannual clinical breast exams to begin at age 20-25, and annual imaging with mammography and /or MRI at the same ages, or 5-10 years prior to the earliest known breast cancer in the family kindred (Gage, 2012). Other cancer types presentation in patients cancer are, sarcoma of soft tissues, gastrointestinal (colon, gastric, pancreatic) cancer, lung cancer, osteosarcoma, hematopoietic cancer such as leukemia and lymphoma, adrenocortical carcinoma, brain tumors. Often is diagnosed in early infancy according to the diagnostic criteria (table 2), and approximately 50% of cases are diagnosed at the age of 30. Families or individuals that do not have all the criteria necessary to the LFS diagnosis have been termed LFS-

Like (LFS-L) (Mai, 2021; Neville, 2001, Thull, 2004, Garber, 2005). For more information about diagnose criteria review: www.nccn.org and www.iarc.fr.

Table 2. Li-Fraumani syndrome and Li-Fraumani-like syndrome Criteria for genetic testing (Mai, 2012)

Classic Li-Fraumani síndrome (LFS)	Patient who developed sarcoma before age 45 and Have a family member in first grade with any type of cancer (< 45 years) and A first or second degree relative with any cancer before 45 years or sarcoma at any age
Li-Fraumani-Like syndrome	**Birch definition:** • A proband with any chils cancer or sarcoma, brain tumor or adrenocortical carcinoma diagnosed before age 45 years and • A first or second degree relative with a typical LFS cancer at any age and • A first or second degree relative with any cancer before age 60 years **Eeles definition:** • Two first or second degree relatives with LFS-related malignancies at any age
Chompret criteria	A proband who has • A tumor belonging to the LFS tumor spectrum (soft tissue sarcoma, osteosarcoma, pre-menopausal breast cancer, brain tumor, adrenocortical carcinoma, leukemia, or bronchoalveolar lung cnacer) before age 46 years and • At least one first or second degree relative with an LFS tumor (expect breast cancer if the proband has breast cancer) before age 56 years or with multiple tumors Or • A proband with multiple tumors (except multiple breast tumors), two of which belong to the LFS tumor spectrum and the first of which occurred before age 46 years Or • A proband who is diagnosed with adrenocortical carcinoma or chorois plexus tumor, irrespective of family history

TP53

In most of families with LFS have been identified germline mutations in *TP53* (*Tumor protein p53*) gene. *TP53* is located in 17p13.1, has 25,767 bases and encode for a protein of 393 amino acids (http://www.genecard.org). *TP53* is a tumor suppression protein, consider it as "*DNA guardian*" for its capacity to identify when cell has a DNA damage, stop the cell cycle in order to repair the DNA and, in case that the damage is major, drive the cell thru apoptosis (Walerych, 2012). *TP53* gene significance has been supported on the others things by the frequent occurrence of breast cancer in LFS patients. In Only the 60-80% of patient with LFS classic has been detectable germline mutation on *TP53,* while patients with LFS-L so not shown detectable *TP53* mutations. The lack of concordance among no *TP53* mutations and the presence of LFS phenotype, can be explained for possible posttranscriptional *TP53* alterations, an complete deletion, the effects of modifier genes, or the possibility of a second locus until now no identified (Malkin, 2011). Additionally *TP53* gene has a higher mutation frequency, higher than any other tumor suppressor gene in human overall. On average, *TP53* is mutated in 31% of all tumors, and in 23% of breast cancer samples, where the principal mutated protooncogene is *PI3KCA* (Walerych, 2012). In some patients had shown germinal mutations on *CHEK2* gene, which encodes for a protein kinase that functions as regulator of the cell cycle, and responds to the damage to the DNA, activating *PT53* and *BRCA1*. In the North of Europe and the United Kingdom, the variant of the gene *CHEK2* 1100delC (deletion of a cytosine at position 1100 of the gene *CHEK)* increases twice the risk for the development of breast cancer in women, and more than ten times in males; In addition to being responsible for 1% of the cases of breast cancer in women and 9% in males. These frequencies are very clear in North America, as it has been the presence of this variant in 0.3% of healthy volunteers, and in 1% of patients with breast cancer; so it is necessary to determine the contribution of the allele *CHEK2* 1100delC, in the development of cancer of the breast (Neville, 2001, Thull, 2004, Garber, 2005).

2. Cowden Syndrome

The Cowden Disease or syndrome of multiple hamartomas (*CS - Cowden syndrome*) (MIM #158350), described by Lloyd and Dennis in 1963, is a rare inherited genodermatosis with an autosomal dominant inheritance pattern and strong predominance of female patients (6:1), which may be fortuitous. CS is associated with both malignant lesions as benign that affect cells of the three germ layers and tissues mostly affected are tissue breast, thyroid, uterus, brain, mucocutaneous tissue and Genitourinary tract. It is estimated that 1 in every 200,000- 250,000 individuals are affected with CS, although this frequency may be underestimated due the difficulty to make the diagnosis; with an age at diagnosis ranging from 13 to 65 years. In this regards, the International Cowden Syndrome Consortium (http://www.nccn.org) established the diagnosis criteria in 2000, where the major (such as breast carcinoma, follicular thyroid carcinoma, multiple gastrointestinal hamartomas, macrocephaly, amog other) and minor criteria (autism spectrum disorder, colon cancer, esophageal glycogenic acanthosis, mental retardation among others) are fundamental at the diagnosis process (Nagy, 2004). The penetrance in CS is related to age, since at the age of 20 years 99% of affected patients present mucocutaneous lesions, which are the most constant and characteristic findings. The risk of breast cancer in patients with CS is 25-50%, represents less than 1% of the cases of breast cancer and occurs between 38 and 46 years of age. Additionally, women with CS have a higher risk (67%) for develop benign breast disease, which include apocrine metaplasia, fibroadenomas, microcysts, adenosis, and hamartoma-like lesions with densely hyalinized collagen (Gage, 2012; Shah, 2012, 2013). Others types of cancer present in patients with CS are the thyroid cancer, typically follicular and papillary occasionally with a risk of 10%, while for cancer endometrial are 5-10%. Due to the high risk for the development of breast cancer, patients with the SC must be monitored from an early age, starting a clinical breast examination before age 25, annual mammogram from 30 years, or in case to have a familiar with CS diagnosis and breast cancer, is important to make the first mammogram 5 years before at the age of diagnosis of breast cancer in the family, as well as an annual physical review beginning at the age of 18 years monitoring lesions in skin and thyroid, inclusive is important to include a thyroid ultrasound. Other important characteristic reported in patients with CS are craniomegaly which is the most commont extracutaneous manifestation (80% incidence), gastrointestinal polyps (approximately 60-85%) with predilection from the esophagus, stomach, and colorectal structures. The small bowel is rarely involved. Polyps are usually small and <5 mm in size; cutaneous fibromas (76%), thyroid abnormalities (62%) and multiple uterine leiomyoma (40%) (Table 3) (Fistarol, 2002; Nagy, 2004; Starink, 1986). According with the mucocutaneous lesions, these include multiple trichilemmomas, oral papillomatosis, facial papules, and acral keratoses. The thrichilemmomas, is defined as a bening hamartomas of the outer sheath of hair follicles, are flesh-colored smooth papules, ranging from 1 -5 mm in size and are present predominantly of the face, head and neck, close to the hairline. Other important mucocutaneous lesions described in CS include the hemangiomas, scrotal and furrowed tonge, neuromas, xanthomas, vitiligo, acanthosis nigricans, perioral and acral lentigines, and frequently the speckled pigmentation of the penis (Shah, 2012, 2013).

PTEN (Phosphatase and Tension Homolog)

In approximately 85% of CS cases has been identified mutations in the *PTEN* (Phosphatase and tensin homolog) gene, which is a gene suppressor turmor located in 10q23.31 (MIM 601728) contains 108,818 bases, 9 exons and encodes for the protein Phosphatidylinositol 3,4,5-triphosphate 3-phosphatase, consists of 403 amino acids and is a member of the super family of genes protein-tyrosine phosphatase (PTP). *PTEN* gene encodes a ubiquitously protein with dual-specificity phosphatase is due to contain a tensin like domain as well as catalytic domain similar to that of the dual specificity protein tyrosine phosphatases. Unlike most of protein tyrosine phosphatases, this protein preferentially dephosphorylates phosphoinositide substrates (www.genecards.org). This activity interferes with the progression of on G1 cell cycle through the negative regulation of PI3-kinase/Akt or PKB signaling pathway. At the same time PTEN protein regulates the mitogen-activated protein kinase (MAPK). Deregulation of these two pathways by *PTEN* inactivation or loss, increased the cell survival and uncontrolled cellular proliferation, resulting in tumor development. The mechanism that gives rise to this syndrome is loss of heterozygosis (LOH) in *PTEN* in 20-60% of cases and is explained with Knudson (double hit hypothesis) hypothesis. In the case of sporadic tumors, both alleles are normal at the moment of the conception, however subsequently have a mutation postzygotic - first hit - in one allele; subsequently a new mutation - second hit - in the other allele causes the LOH, causing a loss in the control of cell growth. In the case of hereditary tumors, the heterozygosity is present from the moment of conception and only a postzygotic mutation is necessary for the LOH (Roman, 2012). Has been reported that germline mutations in *PTEN* gene, is the most common muted gene in several cancers and are associated a number of heritable cancer syndromes, whom collectively are referred to as *PTEN Hamartoma Tumor Syndrome* (PHTS) (Pezzolesi, 2007; Tan, 2012). The PHTS includes the CS,

Bannayan-Riley-Ruvalcaba syndrome [BRRS, (MIM #153480)] and Lhermitte-Duclos syndrome (Romano, 2012). According to the strict diagnostic criteria for CS, 80% of the patients presented germinal mutations in the gene *PTEN,* from which approximately 8.8% of patient are carriers of a germinal mutation and the exons 5, 7, and 8 considering as hot-spots; and all kinds of mutations including deletions, insertions, splice site mutations and large deletions have been identified in these patients. Even though many efforts had been done in order to correlate the different types of cancer or phenotype with the found mutations has not been identified (So, 2012). In such patients, it is important to discard the *Bannayan-Riley-Ruvalcaba* syndrome (MIM-#153480), since certain germinal mutations in *PTEN* have been identified in 60-65% of patients with East syndrome, by what has been considered as an allelic to the CS condition (Neville, 2001, Thull, 2004, Garber, 2005).

3. Peutz-Jeghers Syndrome

Peutz-Jeghers Syndrome *(PJS)* (MIM #175200), is an autosomal dominant condition, which was recognized in 1949 by Jeghers et al. as a localization of intestinal polyposis and pigmentation of the skin and mucous membranes, hence the eponym Peutz- Jeghers syndrome. The PJS has been reported around the world, affecting equally males and females; its estimate incidence is 1:8300 to 1:200,000 live births, and 25% of cases appear to be non familial or sporadic. PJS is caused by germline mutations in the *STK11 (Serine/threonine kinase)* tumor suppressor gene; and characterized by a predisposition (20.3 increased relative risk) to developing malignant tumors in different organs, including stomach, colon, pancreas, intestine thin, thyroid, breast, lung, and uterus. The incidence of cancer in these patients has been estimated at fifteen times higher than in the general population; and the pathognomonic featuresare polyps hamartomatous of the gastrointestinal tract (especially in small intestine), with a specific histology, which may result in symptoms of bleeding or obstruction, being the intussusception a major complication, especially in pediatric patients (Shah, 2012, 2013). Extra-intestinal sites of PJS polyps include kidney, ureter, gallbladder, bronchus and nasal passages. The breast cancer is other important malignance in patient with PJS, affecting at 32% to 54% of patients and being the ductal and occasionally the lobular cancer the more frequent. Recent studies reported that 8% of women with PJS developed breast cancer by age 40, and 32% by age 60 (Gage, 2012; Shah,

2012, 2013). In these cases, it has been observed that the *STK11* gene expression is decreased, which correlates with a histologically high-grade, a large tumor and the presence of metastases to lymph nodes; In addition to partnering with a higher rate of relapse and worse prognosis. More features of the PJS neoplasms are of the genital tract, which include the tumor of sex cord with annular tubules (*SCTAT - Sex cord tumor with annular tubules*), followed in tumor cells of sertoli, Mucinous epithelial tumor, serous tumour and mature teratoma of ovary (Neville, 2001, Thull, 2004). Other characteristic clinical feature is the mucocutaneous hyperpigmentation, which usually is present in childhood as dark macules, and are distributed in the lips and perioral region (94%), hands (74%), buccal mucosa (66%), and feet (62%). However, the mucotutaneous hyperpigmentation also can be present in uncommon region as around the eyes, nostrils, and perianal area. Usually the lesions fade during puberty, with the exception of those on the buccal mucosa (Mishra, 2012). The cumulative risk of any cancer is 67-85% by age 70 and the cumulative risk for CRC is 3% (40 years), 5% (50 years), 15% (60 years), and 39% (70 years). The risk to age 70 for cancers of the pancreas is 11%, utero/ovary/cervix 18%, breast 45% and lung of 17% (Shah, 2012, 2013; Mishra, 2012).

STKT11 Gene

The *STK11* (Serine/Threonine Kinase) gene is the responsible of approximately 70-80% of the PJS; is located in 19.13.3, have 39,029 bases distributes in 10 exons and encode a 433 amino acid protein, STK11 (Liu, 2011). STK11 protein is part of the serine/threonine kinase family and is a well known tumor suppressor, which regulates the activity of AMP-activated protein kinase (AMPK) family members, playing an important role in several processes as cell metabolism, cell polarity, apoptosis and DNA damage response, regulating principally the expression of *p53* gene, as well as its targets genes, such as *p21*. Has been estimated a birth prevalence of mutation in STK11 at 1:25,000 to 1:280,000 (Alexander, 2011; Hemminki, 1998; Liu, 2011).

References

Alexander A, Walker CL. The role of LKB1 and AMPK in cellular responses to stress and damage. *FEBS Lett.* 2011;585(7):952-7.

Antoniou AC, Easton DF. Models of genetic susceptibility to breast cancer. *Oncogene,* 2006b; 25, 5898-5905.

Dumitrescu RG, cotar it I. Understanding breast cancer risk-where do we stand in 2005? *Journal of Cellular Molecular Medicine, 2005*; 9 (1): 208-221.

Evans SC, Lozano G. *The Li-Fraumeni syndrome: an inherited susceptibility to cancer.*

Fistarol SK, Anliker MD, Itin PH. Cowden disease or multiple hamartoma syndrome - cutaneous clue to internal malignancy. *European Journal of Dermatology;* 2002; 12(5): 411-421.

Gage M, Wattendorf D, Henry LR. Translational advances regarding hereditary breast cancer syndromes. *J Surg Oncol.* 2012;105(5):444-451.

Garber JE, Offit K. Hereditary cancer predisposition syndromes. *Journal of Clinical Oncology,* 2005; 23 (2): 276-292.

Glover JN. Insights into the molecular basis of human hereditary breast cancer from studies of the BRCA1 BRCT domain. *Familial cancer,* 2006;5(1):89-93.

Hemminki A, Markie D, Tomlinson I, Avizienyte E, et al. A serine/threonine kinase gene defective in Peutz-Jeghers syndrome. *Nature.* 1998;391(6663):184-7.

Hisada M, Garber JE, Fung CY, Fraumeni JF Jr, Li FP. Multiple primary cancers in families with Li-Fraumeni syndrome. *J Natl Cancer Inst.* 1998;90(8):606-611.

Liu L, Du X, Nie J. A novel de novo mutation in LKB1 gene in a Chinese Peutz Jeghers syndrome patient significantly diminished p53 activity. *Clin Res Hepatol Gastroenterol.* 2011;35(3):221-6.

Mai PL, Malkin D, Garber JE, Schiffman JD, Weitzel JN, et al. Li-Fraumeni syndrome: report of a clinical research workshop and creation of a research consortium. *Cancer Genet.* 2012;205(10):479-487.

Malkin D. Li-fraumeni syndrome. Genes Cancer. 2011;2(4):475-484. *Mol Med Today.* 1997;3(9):390-395.

Nagy R, Sweet K, Eng C. Highly penetrant hereditary cancer syndromes. *Oncogene.* 2004;23(38):6445-6470.

Neville PJ, Morland SJ, Vaziri SAJ, Casey G. The genetics of breast and ovarian cancer. In: Cowell JK (ed). *Molecular genetics of cancer 2nd ed.* 2001:53-80.

Pezzolesi MG, Zbuk KM, Waite KA, Eng C. Comparative genomic and functional analyses reveal a novel cis-acting PTEN regulatory element as a highly conserved functional E-box motif deleted in Cowden syndrome. *Human Molecular Genetic,* 2007; 16: 1058-1071.

Rebecca Nagy, Kevin Sweet and Charis Eng. Highly penetrant hereditary cancer syndromes. *Oncogene;* 2004. 23, 6445-6470.

Romano C and Schepis C. PTEN Gene: A model for Genetics Disease in Dermatology. *The Scientific World Journal;* 2012. 2012: 252457

Shah KR, Boland CR, Patel M, Thrash B, Menter A. Cutaneous manifestations of gastrointestinal disease: part I. *J Am Acad Dermatol.* 2013;68(2):189.

Singletary SE. Rating the risk factors for breast cancer. *Annals of Surgery,* 2003; 237 (4): 474-482.

Starink TM, van der Veen JP, Arwert F, de Waal LP, et al. The Cowden syndrome: a clinical and genetic study in 21 patients. *Clinical Genetic,* 1986; 29 (3): 222-33.

Tan MH, Mester JL, Ngeoe J, et al. Lifetime Cancer Risks in Individuals with Germline PTEN Mutations. *Clin Cancer Res,* 2012; 18: 400-407.

Thull DL, Vogel VG. Recognition and management of hereditary breast cancer syndromes. *The Oncologist;* 2004; 9 (1), 13-24.

Walerych D, Napoli M, Collavin L, Del Sal G. The rebel angel: mutant p53 as the driving oncogene in breast cancer. *Carcinogenesis.* 2012;33(11):2007-2017.

Index

D

N

O

P

Q

R

S

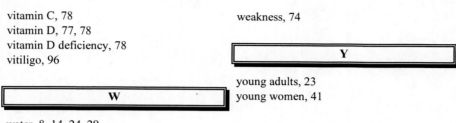